**Fast Facts**

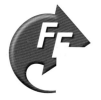

D1646188

# Fast Facts:
# Bipolar Disorder

Second edition

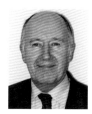

**Guy Goodwin** FMedSci FRCPsych
Professor of Psychiatry
University of Oxford Department of Psychiatry
Warneford Hospital
Oxford, UK

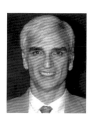

**Gary Sachs** MD
Director, Bipolar Clinic and Research Program
Massachusetts General Hospital and
Associate Professor of Psychiatry
Harvard Medical School
Boston, USA

**Declaration of Independence**
This book is as balanced and as practical as we can make it.
Ideas for improvement are always welcome: feedback@fastfacts.com

HEA

Fast Facts: Bipolar Disorder
First published 2004
Second edition 2010; reprinted February 2

Text © 2010 Guy Goodwin, Gary Sachs
© 2010 in this edition Health Press Limite
Health Press Limited, Elizabeth House, Qı
Oxford OX14 3LN, UK
Tel: +44 (0)1235 523233
Fax: +44 (0)1235 523238

Book orders can be placed by telephone or via the website.
For regional distributors or to order via the website, please go to:
www.fastfacts.com
For telephone orders, please call +44 (0)1752 202301 (UK and Europe),
1 800 247 6553 (USA, toll free), +1 419 281 1802 (Americas) or
+61 (0)2 9698 7755 (Asia–Pacific).

Fast Facts is a trademark of Health Press Limited.

A CIP record for this title is available from the British Library.

ISBN 978-1-905832-52-1

Goodwin G (Guy)
Fast Facts: Bipolar Disorder/
Guy Goodwin, Gary Sachs

Medical illustrations by Dee McLean, London, UK.
Typesetting and page layout by Zed, Oxford, UK.
Printed by Latimer Trend & Company Limited, Plymouth, UK.

Text printed on biodegradable and recyclable paper
manufactured using elemental chlorine free (ECF)
wood pulp from well-managed forests.

FSC

Mixed Sources
Product group from well-managed
forests and other controlled sources
Cert no. SGS-COC-005493
www.fsc.org
© 1996 Forest Stewardship Council

# Glossary

**Affective psychosis:** mental illnesses that are psychotic in form (delusions and hallucinations) but arise in the course of mood disorder. The psychotic features are an expression of the severity of the depressive or manic episodes and their content is strongly colored by the mood.

**Antipsychotic drugs:** medicines that are primarily used to treat psychotic symptoms. Typical antipsychotics, of which the prototype was chlorpromazine, readily produce motor side effects – usually restlessness or rigidity. They are also sometimes called neuroleptics, or major tranquilizers. Atypical antipsychotics have been developed in recent years to reduce the burden of motor side effects. Antipsychotics all antagonize the actions of the neurotransmitter dopamine, and are also antimanic.

**Axis I:** in the recommended diagnostic scheme of the *Diagnostic and Statistical Manual of Mental Disorders*, fourth edition (DSM-IV), illnesses are classified on separate axes, which are independent of each other (as, for example, shape and color might be). Axis I diagnoses are the primary psychiatric disorders such as bipolar I disorder or schizophrenia.

**Axis II:** this other axis of the DSM-IV scheme classifies patients according to lifelong personality characteristics, if these are judged to be extreme – the so-called personality disorders. Personality diagnoses are not very reliable, but they capture something important about extreme personality styles.

**Bipolar:** this term is used to describe a range of illnesses in which there are disturbances of mood into both depression and elation – the poles of affective experience.

**Bipolar I disorder:** a diagnosis that requires a single episode of mania. However, it is the rule that patients who experience mania also experience major depression.

**Bipolar II disorder:** a diagnosis that requires a history of both major depression and hypomania, but no history of mania.

**Bipolar NOS:** bipolar disorder not otherwise specified

**Cognitive–behavior therapy (CBT):** a psychological treatment that derives from the idea that conscious thoughts and explicit beliefs may exacerbate mood or anxiety states. The therapy aims to elicit and question such thoughts and beliefs and to challenge patients to behave differently when they have them, or literally to restructure the way they think. It has a strong tradition of empirical measurement and a better evidence base than most 'talking therapies' or counseling.

**Cognitive impairment:** human cognition can be thought of as a collection of different domains such as attention, memory and executive function. Performance in these different domains can be measured more or less independently and compared with the average for individuals of a given age

4

and education. A person is said to show cognitive impairment when they perform poorly in one or more of these domains. Even small impairments are of interest because they predict difficulty at work, especially for able people.

***Diagnostic and Statistical Manual of Mental Disorders*, fourth edition (DSM-IV):** published by the American Psychiatric Association, DSM-IV lays out simple rules for making psychiatric diagnoses that enable diagnostic reliability to be achieved. These rules – and hence the diagnostic categories – are arbitrary however. They should be thought of as working hypotheses (and may turn out to be false) but nevertheless provide an essential preliminary framework for scientific psychiatry.

**Electroconvulsive therapy (ECT):** a highly effective treatment for severe depression and, probably, for mania. Before the introduction of ECT in the 1930s, the induction of seizures to treat psychosis was performed chemically. The use of electricity was, and to some extent still is, controversial. It is now extremely safe when performed under a brief period of general anesthesia with a neuromuscular blockade to prevent musculoskeletal damage. The main disadvantage is the effects on memory, but some of the complaints made are so extreme that they should be viewed as unexplained medical symptoms.

**Endogenous:** originating from within the body.

**Euthymia:** interludes of normal mood between episodes of depression or mania.

**Exogenous:** having its origins from without (cf: endogenous).

**Extrapyramidal side effects (EPS):** antipsychotics block dopamine neurotransmission in the basal ganglia, which leads to EPS. Acute effects include motor restlessness (akathisia), stiffness/slowing and gait disturbance. These symptoms resemble those seen in Parkinson's disease – a degenerative disease of the dopamine neurons in the basal ganglia. More rarely, antipsychotics provoke acute dystonic reactions – abnormal postures often accompanied by upward staring of the eyes.

**(functional) Magnetic resonance imaging ([f]MRI):** a method based on the magnetization of complex molecules by a strong external magnetic field. The behavior of these molecules can be detected after a test field is briefly turned on. fMRI is a variant of the method that detects changes in the local balance between oxygenated and deoxygenated hemoglobin in the blood. Slightly paradoxically, increased brain activity results in relative hyperperfusion and a greater local concentration of oxygenated hemoglobin.

**Hypomania:** characterized by the presence of mood elevation, usually resulting in increased energy and confidence but without impairment of function (indeed, often the converse – improved attainment).

**Hypothalamic–pituitary–adrenal (HPA) axis:** the secretion of cortisol from the adrenal cortex is controlled by adrenocorticotropic hormone from the pituitary gland; this, in turn, is controlled by corticotropin-releasing hormone, which is secreted by the hypothalamus into the portal pituitary system.

**Index case:** a primary subject in a clinical study. The features of this subject may define how a scale behaves or how heritable a condition is within the families of 'index cases'.

**Mania:** a mental state of extreme mood elevation or irritability that is accompanied by characteristic changes in behavior and impairment of normal personal or social function. There may be associated psychotic features.

**Pharmacokinetic:** effects on drug action caused by changes in drug availability (or drug levels) – for example, because of changes in drug metabolism or absorption.

**Placebo:** inert tablets that are matched so that they appear identical to an active comparator. Positive placebo effects are common in trials of psychotropic medicines. In other words, groups of patients given placebo show large reductions in symptoms. These effects arise from a number of mechanisms that have nothing to do with the placebo, such as exaggerated baseline scores, regression to the mean and spontaneous recovery. The small effects literally due to the placebo may result from the positive attribution of change to the supposed action of the tablet – a cognitive mechanism.

**Psychomotor retardation:** the obvious slowing of speech, gesture and thought that accompanies severe depression.

**Psychosis:** the traditional term for mental states characterized by delusions and/or hallucinations. The loss of contact with reality makes patients more likely to be vulnerable or dangerous.

**Randomized controlled trial:** a clinical experiment in which patients are assigned at random to two or more different treatment groups; the outcomes are compared with the control group (e.g. those receiving placebo or the current 'gold standard' therapy).

**Rapid cycling:** an illness course in which discrete episodes of depression or mood elevation occur four or more times per year (*also see* ultrarapid cycling).

**Schizophrenia:** a chronic relapsing illness characterized by bizarre delusions, auditory hallucinations, disorganized thinking and, frequently, social withdrawal/isolation; different from bipolar disorder because of the relative absence of extremes of mood and the worse social outcome.

**Tardive dyskinesia:** the abnormal involuntary movement disorder associated with long-term use of typical antipsychotic drugs. It generally involves spontaneous movement of the lips and face, and arises after prolonged treatment (usually years).

**Ultrarapid cycling:** unlike rapid cycling (above) there is no universally accepted definition for this term. It can be informally applied to an illness course in which episodes occur every few days (perhaps 12 or more times per year). Distinct abrupt mood shifts of less than 24 hours' duration may be defined as ultra-ultra rapid or ultradian cycling.

**Unipolar disorder:** the experience of only one pole of mood disorder. In practice, this diagnosis can apply only to depression – major depressive disorder – because DSM-IV defines bipolar disorder with reference only to mania. Unipolar mania is, however, extremely rare.

# Introduction

Bipolar disorder, formerly known as manic depression, is a disease with a long history. In antiquity, Greek clinicians described both the euphoria and psychosis associated with manic states, and the despair and suicidal inclinations associated with melancholia, the older word for depression. However, the great distinction between 'manic-depressive insanity' and the other major form of functional psychosis – dementia praecox or schizophrenia – was first made explicitly by Emil Kraepelin in the late 19th century. Like other psychiatrists at the time, his observations were confined to the clientele of asylums. Therefore, he saw the worst cases of affective disorder and its most extreme manifestations in psychotic depression or mania.

Kraepelin did not distinguish between patients with both elevation and depression of mood and those who showed only psychotic but unipolar depression. The emphasis on bipolarity is modern and arose from the work of Angst and Perris in the 1960s. It is the distinction that they drew between bipolar and unipolar cases that now highlights mania and mood elevation as the defining feature of bipolar disorder.

A central feature of the Kraepelinian dichotomy between affective psychosis and schizophrenia was the difference that he discerned in the

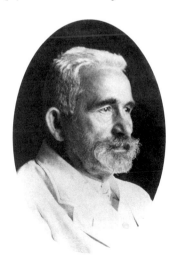

**Figure 1** Emil Kraepelin (1856–1926) first made the distinction between 'manic-depressive insanity' and other forms of psychosis. Source: The Wellcome Library, London.

outcomes of the two conditions. The outcome in schizophrenia he saw as being consistent: often being poor with residual symptoms, cognitive impairments and social withdrawal. By contrast, bipolar disorder is compatible with complete recovery, although we also know that this is the exception rather than the rule. Outcomes, and the need to improve them, are one of the major reasons why the treatment of bipolar disorder must be moved forward.

Bipolar disorder has been a neglected disease, certainly by comparison with schizophrenia, although we believe that this is now changing. We have a better understanding of the prevalence and neurobiology of bipolar disorder, as the advances of the last 2 decades have been applied to psychiatric disorders. Bipolar disorder is no longer a rare disorder seen only by psychiatrists working with psychotic inpatients. Statements that may be true for more severe examples of the illness may not ring so true for the milder range of bipolar diagnoses. Furthermore, treatment has improved as researchers have explored the illness as a target for new classes of medicines, and interest in formal psychological interventions for bipolar disorder is growing. In parallel with these essentially scientific advances, there has been a much greater appreciation of the plight of patients with the illness, the impact it has on their lives and the many failures, big and small, of the services

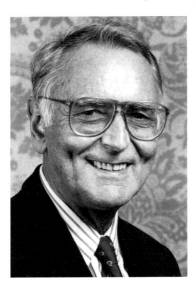

**Figure 2** Jules Angst has played a major role in increasing our understanding of the diagnosis and course of bipolar disorder.

provided to help them. The emphasis on patient self-management is more fundamental than for almost any other illness of which we have experience. The individual patient must become expert in their own condition. The need for a genuinely collaborative and mutually educative doctor–patient relationship in bipolar disorder has the potential to inform practice in many areas of medicine.

These relatively recent developments have paved the way for a much more unified view of the illness worldwide, and have facilitated clearer agreement on the vital research agenda for the next decade. We have had the privilege of participating in the development of this consensus and planning for future studies.

This book provides a brief synopsis of current understanding and strategies. We hope it will be of interest to anyone whose mission is to treat patients with bipolar disorder and to champion their cause. This includes primary care physicians with an interest in the disorder, psychiatrists, therapists, nurses and medical students, all of whom can provide so much help to individual patients in their care.

Finally, we hope that patients and their families will use this book. They can provide the ultimate stimulus to improve practice by directly challenging their doctors to keep up to date and alert to new developments. We hope they will also participate enthusiastically in research into the causes and nature of bipolar disorder, and the randomized trials that can improve its treatment.

# 1 Definitions: diagnosis and comorbidity

The lasting contribution of investigators in the 20th century has been to formalize the criteria by which psychiatric diagnoses are made. The *Diagnostic and Statistical Manual of Mental Disorders*, fourth edition (DSM-IV), which includes the latest revisions to these criteria, gives clear and explicit rules for diagnosing bipolar disorder. Such diagnoses are sometimes criticized for their lack of validity. In fact, their strength lies in their reliability, which allows us to be confident that when we describe bipolar disorder we are describing something that others could recognize in their own practice or experience.

Diagnosis is a fundamental activity for doctors. It implies that there has been application of a medical model. We believe that the medical model is useful in diagnosing bipolar disorder – indeed, we cannot see a viable or reliable alternative. However, by a medical model, we mean a unifying scientific discipline, not an exclusive reliance on medicines. This point is important to us and we return to it in Chapter 4.

## Mania

The diagnosis of mania depends on the recognition of key symptoms (Table 1.1), which must either be present for at least 1 week or have resulted in hospital admission. Manic symptoms result in severe impairment of the normal ability to function; this is the additional criterion that defines mania in the absence of admission to hospital. Mania varies in severity from severe psychotic exhaustion to a mischievous state of elation accompanied by very bad judgment.

Manic states must always be taken seriously because of the potential for patients to do themselves irreparable physical harm by taking risks, especially when driving, or social harm from imprudence, excessive spending or sexual indiscretions. It is almost always essential to recognize the disorder and initiate treatment as soon as possible.

Psychotic features are relatively common in mania and, according to most surveys, are seen in about 50% of cases. Psychosis usually manifests as delusions that are mood congruent: they are often

TABLE 1.1

**DSM-IV criteria for mania (mania defines bipolar I disorder)**

The core symptoms must be present for 1 week and/or require hospital admission.

1  A distinct period of abnormally and persistently elevated, expansive or irritable mood, lasting at least 1 week (or any duration if hospitalization is necessary)

2  During the period of mood disturbance, three (or more) of the following symptoms have persisted (four if the mood is only irritable) and have been present to a significant degree:

   a  inflated self-esteem or grandiosity

   b  decreased need for sleep (e.g. feels rested after only 3 hours of sleep)

   c  more talkative than usual or pressure to keep talking

   d  flight of ideas or subjective experience that thoughts are racing

   e  distractibility (i.e. attention too easily drawn to unimportant or irrelevant external stimuli)

   f  increase in goal-directed activity (socially, at work or school, or sexually) or psychomotor agitation

   g  excessive involvement in pleasurable activities that have a high potential for painful consequences (e.g. engaging in unrestrained buying sprees, sexual indiscretions or foolish business investments)

3  The symptoms do not meet the criteria for a 'mixed episode'

4  The mood disturbance is sufficiently severe to cause marked impairment in occupational functioning or in usual social activities or relationships with others, or to necessitate hospitalization to prevent harm to self or others, or there are psychotic features

5  The symptoms are not due to the direct physiological effects of a substance (e.g. a drug of misuse, a medication or other treatment) or a general medical condition (e.g. hyperthyroidism)

grandiose, reflecting the elevation of mood, and may, for example, overestimate the personal qualities of the patient with regard to their attractiveness, ability and power. Some patients with mania show mood-incongruent symptoms – delusions and hallucinations similar to those seen in schizophrenia. All the features of schizophrenia can coexist with mania. The diagnosis of bipolar disorder remains if the psychotic features resolve along with the abnormal mood state, but this is then considered an affective psychosis. The DSM-IV defines schizoaffective disorder as a condition in which patients experience episodes that meet the full criteria for mania or depression along with psychosis, and experience persistence of the psychotic symptoms after resolution of the abnormal mood state. Other classification systems use the term 'schizoaffective' to describe states that include a combination of the two recognized syndromes.

Bipolar I disorder in DSM-IV is diagnosed on the basis of mania alone, although there is often a history of depression and certainly a risk of future depression. However, the course of the illness is not individually predictable.

## Hypomania

Functional impairment underpins a crucial distinction between mania and hypomania made in DSM-IV. Hypomania is not associated with significant functional impairment and may be viewed by patients as positively desirable. This state is arbitrarily required to last 4 days or more to meet the DSM-IV diagnostic criteria.

A state of hypomania may be the prelude to mania in bipolar I disorder, or it may be the only elevation in mood that an individual ever experiences. In the former case it is an indication for vigilance and usually also for active treatment to avoid mania. Hypomania in a patient with major depression constitutes a diagnosis of bipolar II disorder.

Bipolar II disorder is assuming increasing importance because it is rather prevalent, if hitherto often undiagnosed, among patients presenting with depression. Unfortunately, hypomania is not yet a familiar diagnosis to many clinicians. Patients seldom complain of hypomania and, moreover, the term is widely misused – almost out of a sense of politeness – to describe mania. Failure to detect hypomania will, of course, render clinicians oblivious to the existence of bipolar II disorder, which will usually present as major depression.

## Mixed states

The classic view of mania emphasizes euphoria, expansiveness and overactivity. There are, however, states of mania that are much more a mixture of manic and depressive features. A particular additional risk with such illnesses is suicide, which almost always correlates with depressive symptoms.

The recognition of mixed states may pose significant diagnostic problems even for experienced psychiatrists, because presentations are difficult to classify as recognizable vignettes. The two most common forms are rapidly alternating mania and depression, or a severe depression with complete absence of euphoria or humor but showing labile periods of pressured, irritable hostility and paranoia.

## Major depression

The depressions associated with bipolar disorder have much in common with those experienced by patients with other types of depressive illness. The diagnostic criteria for major depression in DSM-IV require that five or more of the key symptoms are present for more than 2 weeks. As shown in Table 1.2, there are many key symptoms and therefore many ways of becoming depressed.

On average, certain features are more common in bipolar than unipolar disorders. Marked psychomotor retardation is more common, together with psychotic depression in younger people and atypical features of depression, such as hypersomnia. Patients may describe such extreme loss of energy, motivation and interest that it feels physical in its intensity. This can make recognition of early episodes of depression in bipolar disorder more difficult than in unipolar cases. Patients will often describe 'not knowing' what such episodes were. Paradoxically, the more subjectively obvious experience of milder depression may be easier to recognize and describe. A first-degree relative with bipolar depression should also suggest a bipolar diagnosis in a patient with major depression.

Depression is usually the predominant abnormality of mood and an important cause of functional impairment in patients with bipolar disorder, and contributes to their increased mortality from suicide.

TABLE 1.2
**DSM-IV criteria for major depression**

Five (or more) of the following symptoms have been present during the same 2-week period and represent a change from previous functioning; at least one of the symptoms is either (1) depressed mood or (2) loss of interest or pleasure. Note: do not include symptoms that are clearly due to a general medical condition, or mood-incongruent delusions or hallucinations.

1 Depressed mood most of the day, nearly every day, as indicated by either subjective report (e.g. feels sad or empty) or observation made by others (e.g. appears tearful); note: in children and adolescents, can be irritable mood

2 Markedly diminished interest or pleasure in all, or almost all, activities most of the day, nearly every day (as indicated by either subjective account or observation made by others)

3 Significant weight loss when not dieting, or weight gain (e.g. a change of more than 5% of bodyweight in a month), or decrease or increase in appetite nearly every day; in children, consider failure to make expected weight gains

4 Insomnia or hypersomnia nearly every day

5 Psychomotor agitation or retardation nearly every day (observable by others, not merely subjective feelings of restlessness or being slowed down)

6 Fatigue or loss of energy nearly every day

7 Feelings of worthlessness or excessive or inappropriate guilt (which may be delusional) nearly every day (not merely self-reproach or guilt about being sick)

8 Diminished ability to think or concentrate, or indecisiveness, nearly every day (either by subjective account or as observed by others)

9 Recurrent thoughts of death (not just fear of dying), recurrent suicidal ideation without a specific plan, or a suicide attempt or a specific plan for committing suicide

## Minor bipolar disorder

Bipolar I and II disorders are broadly accepted categories in DSM-IV. Other generally less severe manifestations of mood elevation and depression are now also thought to merit recognition as bipolar disorder. Bipolar disorder not otherwise specified (bipolar NOS) is a DSM-IV category that includes any of the following:

- recurrent subthreshold hypomania in the presence of intercurrent major depression
- recurrent hypomania (at least two episodes) in the absence of recurrent major depression with or without subthreshold major depression
- recurrent subthreshold hypomania in the absence of intercurrent major depression with or without subthreshold major depression.

The number of symptoms required for a determination of subthreshold hypomania is reduced to two from the DSM-IV requirement of three (or four if the mood is only irritable) to retain the core features of hypomania in the subthreshold definition.

These states are of interest because they may be harbingers of the major syndromes, and they can offer clues to the etiology, particularly heritability. Patients with such symptoms are also increasingly seeking advice. It is a challenge for psychiatry that its core diagnoses, such as bipolar I disorder, do not have qualitative boundaries with milder states. Medicine is traditionally more comfortable with diseases that behave like acute infections.

## Rapid cycling

Patients with four or more episodes of mania, hypomania, mixed states or depression in the preceding 12 months are described as rapid cycling. This definition includes patients who show remission between these episodes and those who cycle continuously (or switch continually) from one polarity to the other without euthymia. The lifetime risk of rapid cycling is around 16%; it persists indefinitely in only a few patients.

Rapid cycling is weakly associated with female sex, bipolar II disorder, current hypothyroidism and a less robust response to lithium (especially the depressive component). It may often be difficult to treat. Rapid cycling may be preceded by exposure to antidepressants and worsened by treatment with antidepressants, but there is no proof of a causal relationship. It is rare for patients to exhibit sustained rapid cycling over periods longer than 2 years. A history of rapid cycling does, however, appear to be a marker of a high propensity to relapse.

No treatment has demonstrated efficacy superior to placebo for control of rapid cycling in patients with bipolar I disorder.

## Comorbidity

Patients with bipolar disorder often also meet the criteria for other psychiatric diagnoses, of which the most important are anxiety-related disorders and substance misuse. These disorders occur much more frequently than might be expected from the rates in the general population.

**Anxiety disorder.** As many as 93% of patients with bipolar I disorder may have an anxiety disorder at some stage in their life. This is such a high figure that anxiety symptoms may be viewed as part of the bipolar phenotype. Anxiety disorders encountered in bipolar patients include, in descending order of prevalence: panic, generalized anxiety disorder and obsessive–compulsive disorder.

Anxiety symptoms or syndromes are sometimes the earliest symptoms that a patient experiences and they may be the most persistent and pervasive. They are clinically most salient between acute episodes and in bipolar depression, though many patients describe anxiety as a component of their manic experience as well, particularly as a prodrome. Indeed, anxiety symptoms may sometimes be the chief determinant of clinical outcome. The presence of comorbid anxiety disorders is associated with earlier age of onset, shorter intervals of wellness, greater substance misuse and higher frequency of suicide attempts.

**Substance misuse** is also a common and clinically significant comorbidity of bipolar I and II disorders. It may be driven in part by the potential of addictive drugs to relieve anxiety and elevate mood. Appropriate assessment and effective treatment of significant substance or alcohol misuse is important because it can improve compliance and bipolar outcomes.

Compulsive behavior may also link substance misuse and overeating. Obesity is a major problem in North America and is increasing in many other parts of the world. Patients with bipolar disorder appear to be particularly prone to obesity. Interestingly, there appears to be a trade-off between alcohol misuse and obesity in that the rates of each were negatively correlated in a large Canadian sample.

'Impulse control' disorders are commonly found in community surveys of bipolar disorder. These include attention deficit hyperactivity disorder, oppositional disorder, intermittent explosive disorder and conduct disorder. The rates of comorbidity in bipolar I disorder are given as around 40% for each disorder. The clinical significance, and implications for treatment, of disorders usually diagnosed in children are not well established for adults.

## Drug-induced psychosis

A drug-induced psychosis (as defined in DSM-IV) should either disappear with clearance of the offending drug or be a transient phenomenon of drug withdrawal. This is quite a restrictive diagnosis. Unfortunately, the term is often used in clinical practice whenever mania is associated with the use of a variety of stimulant drugs. If manic states are sustained, a diagnosis of 'drug-induced psychosis' is likely to be wrong and misleading. Even if a stimulant drug appears to have acted as a trigger, the diagnosis of bipolar disorder is likely to be more appropriate.

Prescribed medications, most commonly levodopa and corticosteroids, are also associated with secondary mania. Thyroid disease, multiple sclerosis, HIV infection or any lesion(s) involving subcortical or cortical areas may similarly be a cause of secondary mania and should be considered in the differential diagnosis. An underlying physical diagnosis is most likely in mature patients with a late onset of mood symptoms.

Antidepressant-induced mania describes a causal relationship between medication use and the occurrence of mania. The presumed causal connection with antidepressants has been hard to prove, as an irregular course of highs and lows is typical for bipolar disorder and nearly all bipolar patients have been exposed to antidepressant medications. Antidepressants may be a trigger for mania and hypomania. This issue is discussed at length in Chapter 6, which covers short-term treatments, but it is also a problem for diagnosis. In DSM-IV, mania or hypomania induced by antidepressants is not regarded as diagnostic of bipolar disorder. The diagnosis can, of course, be made if a patient has had a manic episode while off medicines – but what of patients who switch to mania or hypomania only when prescribed antidepressants? DSM-IV excludes basing a diagnosis of bipolar I or II disorder on episodes attributed to antidepressant treatment, although it leaves open the bipolar NOS designation. However, this is likely to be revised in the fifth edition of the DSM to recognize a bipolar diagnosis in these patients too. Irrespective of labels, the approach to patients who have had treatment-emergent mania should certainly follow the principles we describe for bipolar patients who meet DSM-IV criteria.

## Personality disorder

In DSM-IV, personality disorder may be an 'axis II' accompaniment of any 'axis I' psychiatric diagnosis (axis I and II are defined in the glossary). Accordingly, a diagnosis of bipolar I disorder may be made in someone also judged to have a personality disorder. However, the behavioral disturbances of young people with manic mood elevation pose a particular challenge. If they are interpreted as personality based, not illness based, the 'personality disorder' diagnosis may blind the clinician to bipolar disorder. Failure to diagnose bipolar disorder is a far greater disservice to the patient than 'missing' the personality disorder.

Borderline personality disorder is defined by criteria that include 'mood swings', deliberate self-harm and relationship difficulties, but it requires onset of these symptoms as a constant feature before 18 years of age. A diagnosis of personality disorder cannot, of course, be established by the assessment of behavior during the acute phases of bipolar illness. The possible overlap between borderline symptoms, bipolar spectrum and ultrarapid-cycling bipolar disorder remains uncertain.

Well-validated but purely descriptive personality measures do not yield DSM-IV diagnoses. These scales do, however, suggest a personality signature that differs somewhat from population norms. On the NEO five-factor personality inventory, individuals with bipolar disorder have, on average, significantly higher scores for neuroticism and openness and significantly lower scores for extraversion, agreeableness and conscientiousness compared with the general population. Among patients with mood disorders, higher scores for openness differentiate bipolar from unipolar disorder.

Diagnosis sets the scene for the important questions: what are these mood disorders, why do people develop abnormal mood states and what should we try to do about them?

---

**Key points – definitions: diagnosis and comorbidity**

- DSM-IV provides the preferred framework for the diagnosis of bipolar disorders.
- Mania defines bipolar I disorder.
- Bipolar II disorder is defined by hypomania that is not associated with significant functional impairment, together with major depression.
- Major depression is similar in unipolar and bipolar patients, though psychosis, motor retardation and atypical features should suggest a diagnosis of bipolar disorder, as should a first-degree relative with bipolar disorder.
- Suicide is an important lifelong risk for patients with bipolar disorder.
- Briefer, less severe mood elevations are also described in patients with depression and are currently extending our concept of the bipolar spectrum.
- Hypomania or mania induced by antidepressants or stimulants usually implies a bipolar diagnosis.
- Anxiety and substance or alcohol misuse are the most common significant clinical comorbidities that negatively affect outcome.
- Personality disorders cannot be assessed from behavior during acute episodes.
- Purely descriptive personality measures may be useful for assessing bipolar disorder and planning treatment.

---

## Key references

American Psychiatric Association. *Diagnostic and Statistical Manual for Mental Disorders (DSM-IV)*. Washington, DC: American Psychiatric Association, 1994.

Blader JC, Carlson GA. Increased rates of bipolar disorder diagnoses among U.S. child, adolescent, and adult inpatients, 1996–2004. *Biol Psychiatry* 2007;62:107–14.

Cassidy F, Forest K, Murry E, Carroll BJ. A factor analysis of the signs and symptoms of mania. *Arch Gen Psychiatry* 1998;55:27–32.

Goodwin GM. Hypomania – what's in a name? *Br J Psychiatry* 2002;181:94–5.

Kendell RE. Diagnosis and classification of functional psychoses. *Br Med Bull* 1987;43:499–513.

McIntyre RS, McElroy SL, Konarski JZ et al. Substance use disorders and overweight/obesity in bipolar I disorder: preliminary evidence for competing addictions. *J Clin Psychiatry* 2007;68:1352–7.

Merikangas KR, Akiskal HS, Angst J et al. Lifetime and 12-month prevalence of bipolar spectrum disorder in the National Comorbidity Survey replication. *Arch Gen Psychiatry* 2007;64:543–52.

Mitchell PB, Goodwin GM, Johnson GF, Hirschfeld RMA. Diagnostic guidelines for bipolar depression: a probabilistic approach. *Bipolar Disord* 2008;10:144–52.

Otto MW, Simon NM, Wisniewski SR et al. Prospective 12-month course of bipolar disorder in out-patients with and without comorbid anxiety disorders. *Br J Psychiatry* 2006;189:20–5.

## Genetics

After establishing their name, it is said that the second question asked of all new patients seen at the Maudsley Hospital (London, UK) in the last 60 years has been "Are you a twin?" If you are a twin with any illness, then whether or not your brother or sister is also affected provides vital information about whether or not the condition is inherited. Identical twins share 100% of their genes, while non-identical twins share 50%. Thus, the risk of any inherited illness or trait also being expressed in the co-twin is higher in monozygotic pairs than in dizygotic pairs. In the case of severe bipolar I disorder, the risk has been estimated to be as high as 80%; in other words, the disorder is highly heritable.

Bipolar disorder therefore runs in families. Furthermore, diagnoses that are related in a genetic sense to bipolar disorder may also appear at an increased rate in families. When the risks of illnesses in first-degree relatives of index cases are studied, it is found that the risk of bipolar disorder in the families of bipolar patients is about 6% compared with about 0.5% in the general population. The risk of psychosis (usually schizophrenia) is similarly increased in the relatives of patients with schizophrenia (Figure 2.1). Figure 2.1 also shows the unexpected finding that the risk of unipolar depression is increased approximately equally in the families of index cases with schizophrenia, bipolar or unipolar disorder. In addition, there may be some increase in the risk of psychosis in patients with bipolar disorder.

If we think of these different diagnoses as being largely correlated with individual genes or groups of genes, it seems that the phenotype of bipolar disorder is associated not just with 'bipolar genes' but also with genes for unipolar depression (common in relatives) and genes for psychosis (with psychotic phenotypes being encountered in relatives at a much lower frequency). Index cases with schizoaffective disorder have an excess of both bipolar disorder and psychosis among their relatives (not shown in Figure 2.1), which is what would be predicted if such cases have the genes predisposing to both disorders.

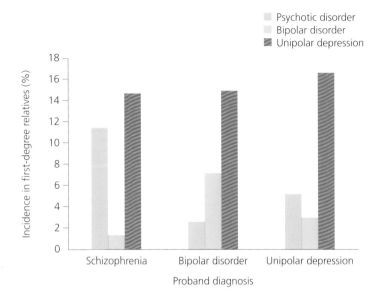

Psychotic disorder
Bipolar disorder
Unipolar depression

**Figure 2.1** Frequencies of different diagnoses in the families of patients with different index illnesses. A patient with schizophrenia will have more family members with psychosis than bipolar disorder; the converse is the case for a patient with bipolar disorder. Notice the increased risk of major depression in the family members of patients with schizophrenia, bipolar disorder or unipolar depression. Modified from Gershon ES et al. 1982.

This suggests that bipolar disorder is a complex phenotype and inheritance is likely to be determined by a number of functionally related genes, as illustrated schematically in Figure 2.2. This has turned out to be the case in most relatively common somatic diseases as well. The identity of these genes is being established as more and more detailed genetic analyses are being applied to larger and larger samples. We do not find, and indeed we would not expect to find, clear evidence for single-gene inheritance or genome scans suggesting single loci homogeneously related to bipolar disorder in reasonably sized samples. Instead, the hunt is for genes of quite small effect, some of which may contribute to a risk for depression, others of which may contribute specifically to a risk for mania or psychosis. There appear to be statistically significant associations between bipolar disorder and

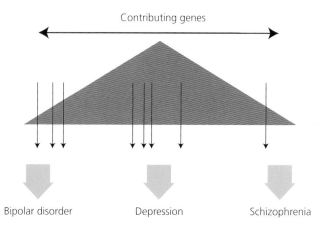

**Figure 2.2** Illustration of the polygenic inheritance of bipolar disorder. The red triangle represents a spectrum of functionally related genes that together may contribute to a range of psychiatric disorders (shown as green arrows). The vertical lines represent polymorphic genes that may act in a single individual to produce bipolar disorder. The numbers of genes that make up the relevant genes and the actual numbers required for illness to arise are unknown, but may be large.

polymorphisms in genes coding for ankyrin G and the alpha chain of L-type calcium channels.

These results merely identify vulnerability factors in populations and are of no practical significance for individual diagnoses. Indeed, the predictive values of tests for the alleles associated with bipolar disorder are so low as to negate the value of testing.

Mania, depression and schizophrenia can only show the variation that they do if a mix of genetic factors are involved. It is now obvious that the many genes already implicated as increasing the risk for common psychiatric disorders leave plenty of scope for heterogeneity. Thus, several of the early genes to be reliably implicated in schizophrenia are also positive for psychotic features in bipolar disorder. Interestingly, the list of genes so far implicated has not identified the monoamine receptors, where current medicines tend to act (see below).

Instead, the genes often encode proteins believed to be involved in regulating the transcription of other genes and cellular adhesion. They look more like the instructions for brain development than for brain function as currently understood. The challenge is to tease out the functions of individual genes or groups of genes acting in development or in relevant neuronal systems to 'cause' the phenotypes we call schizophrenia or bipolar I disorder.

Heritability is not just an issue for clinical scientists. It matters a great deal to patients with bipolar disorder and their families. In the most common case, in which the spouse of the person with bipolar disorder has no history of mood disorder, the risk of their child being affected is of the order of 6%. This can be expressed in a frightening way as representing a 12-fold increase in risk over the general population rate of 0.5% or, less alarmingly, as a 1 in 17 chance that the child will have bipolar disorder. Both expressions of risk are correct, but the latter is probably what matters most for the patient and family. Of course, other unions may give rise to higher risks, especially if both parents have mood disorders or come from families in which severe mood disorder is prominent.

## Neurobiology

To say that bipolar disorder is largely determined by genes is currently a true, but trite, statement. It is known that genes code for proteins and that proteins make up the enzymes, receptors and intracellular signals released by receptor activation on which the neurotransmitters act in the brain. Genes also control neuronal growth and development. The environmental experience of a developing nervous system feeds back and may modify or fix the versions of genes that are active in development. There are therefore myriad ways in which genetic variation could have an impact on a mature nervous system.

In the case of bipolar disorder, and unlike schizophrenia, there is little evidence for an environmental trigger factor or a neurodevelopmental defect. Most children who will develop bipolar disorder appear to reach adulthood without showing obvious developmental, behavioral or temperamental abnormalities. It is, however, too early to say that there will be no important measurable behavioral variations associated with bipolar disorder; this is currently an area of active investigation (see below).

It is commonly supposed that most severe mental illnesses have a trigger. Most cases of depression, for example, are preceded by life events. This is also true of the first onset of schizophrenic psychoses, but to a lesser extent. While less studied, the onset of mania may also be weakly associated with a life event or events, although not clearly 'negative' ones. However, because life events are common in young people and bipolar disorder starts at a young age, the specificity of this relationship is difficult to establish. A trigger may sometimes initiate an episode, but it is never sufficient to cause mania in the absence of a vulnerable phenotype. Triggers have the same relationship to the real causes of severe bipolar disorder as a spark has to gunpowder. The persistent finding of hypothalamic–pituitary–adrenal (HPA) axis dysfunction in mood disorder may eventually explain how 'social' stressors can be represented as physiological constructs.

How acute states of mood disturbance develop on a background of euthymia remains uncertain. Many studies have described biological abnormalities in depression and to a lesser extent in mania, but the findings barely add up to a coherent theory. Acute states of mania and depression produce profound disturbances of physiology and behavior, so perhaps it is no surprise that many systems are found to be perturbed in some way. Unfortunately, such changes may be epiphenomena. It is much more interesting when any biological abnormality is found that characterizes the euthymic condition and gives a basis for understanding the vulnerability to relapse that typifies the disorder.

## Psychopharmacology

Greater understanding of the neurobiology of manic or depressive states would provide candidate systems in which to look for the predicted genetic effects. The greatest clues to the etiology have come from the toxic effects of stimulants and the fortuitous discovery of medicines that seem to be effective in treating common psychiatric symptoms.

**Mania.** There are many similarities between manic states and the changes that take place in volunteers given euphoriant doses of amphetamine. In both cases, there is an elevation in mood and energy and a reduced need for sleep. It is therefore curious that the 'dopamine hypothesis' is usually associated with schizophrenia, depending as it does on the less common psychotomimetic effects of amphetamine. Amphetamine provokes a state that more reliably corresponds to mania than to schizophrenia. This places excess release of monoamines, especially dopamine, as a central mechanism that possibly underlies the psychopathology of mania. Studies of transmitter metabolites in cerebrospinal fluid support the idea of increased neurotransmitter turnover in mania.

The central role of dopamine overactivity in mania is supported by the now very convincing evidence that atypical antipsychotics, all of which occupy the dopamine $D_2$ receptor, are effective antimanic agents (see Chapter 6). In addition, depletion of the substrates for dopamine synthesis (the amino acids tyrosine and phenylalanine) attenuates the effects of amphetamine in animals and humans, and is also antimanic. Some aspects of the cognitive performance of manic individuals, such as increased distractibility on performing tasks requiring attention, may also be related to excess dopamine function. The relevant neuroanatomy lies in the connections that exist between the striatum and the frontal cortex, and possibly the direct projections of dopamine neurons to the frontal cortex (Figure 2.3).

Dopamine may not, however, offer a complete explanation for mania. Mania is also treated with lithium, and relapse can be reliably triggered by lithium withdrawal. The pharmacology of lithium influences dopamine function only indirectly. It has also long been known that glutamate is the predominant excitatory neurotransmitter in the central nervous system. Several reports have associated elevated brain glutamate with acute mania.

**Depression.** Contemporary ideas about depression have been strongly influenced by our understanding of serotonergic function in the brain. When the availability of the serotonin substrate tryptophan is depleted by loading with other amino acids, recovered individuals with recurrent unipolar depression show a return of depressive symptoms. Such observations suggest a very strong and direct link between serotonin

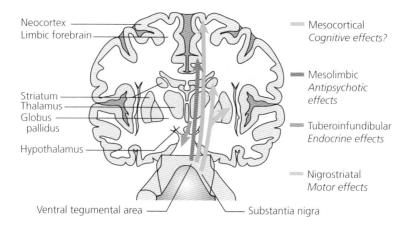

Neocortex
Limbic forebrain

Striatum
Thalamus
Globus
pallidus
Hypothalamus

Ventral tegumental area

Substantia nigra

Mesocortical
*Cognitive effects?*

Mesolimbic
*Antipsychotic
effects*

Tuberoinfundibular
*Endocrine effects*

Nigrostriatal
*Motor effects*

**Figure 2.3** The connections that exist between the striatum and the frontal cortex, and possibly the direct projections of the dopamine neurons to the frontal cortex, may be relevant to the role of dopamine in attention and reward. The globus pallidus is concerned with motor activity, and the projections to the pituitary exert inhibitory control over the release of prolactin.

function in the brain and the risk of depression in vulnerable subjects. By contrast, efforts to demonstrate symptom return after depletion of tryptophan in patients with bipolar I disorder have failed. It therefore remains uncertain whether serotonin has a similarly fundamental role in the biology of bipolar depression as it appears to have in unipolar cases. It could, and probably does, still provide a pathway for treatment, because selective serotonin-reuptake inhibitors appear to be effective in bipolar depression.

Norepinephrine (noradrenaline) rivals serotonin for the attention of neuroscientists interested in depression. Its depletion may also result in depression under some circumstances. Patients who have recovered from acute episodes of mania or depression show a pattern of cognitive impairment that is compatible with a noradrenergic deficit. It is possible that some noradrenergic projections are impaired by repeated episodes of major depression and/or mania, resulting in an increased risk of depression and an enduring deficit of sustained attention.

**Psychopathology and neuroscience.** Interest in the neurobiology of emotion has increased in recent years. It is now possible to study the behavioral and neural basis for emotion processing in humans using appropriate tests of emotional bias in attention, perception and memory. Imaging, particularly the availability of non-invasive functional magnetic resonance imaging (fMRI), has made the localization of underlying neural processes relatively routine. These methods are being used in many centers to explore bipolar disorder. It is already clear that the emotional bias that is evident in the symptoms of depression or mania is reflected in the processing biases that are evident when individuals view different facial expressions or make emotional choices. The next stage is to apply such tests to appropriately chosen individuals before they develop bipolar disorder and so determine whether such biases in emotional processing exist before the first episode and therefore constitute the substrate of their risk to develop the condition.

This approach is attractive because it provides a description of the underlying neural processing that is inherently translational. In other words, it has the potential to inform the development of medicines or psychological treatments that could prevent the development of new episodes of illness.

## Endocrine function

There is a persistent, but not entirely consistent, theme of disturbed endocrine function in mood disorder, including bipolar disorder. Raised cortisol output is observed in severe depression and mania but tends to normalize on recovery. The meaning of this phenomenon is still uncertain. The HPA axis can be tested by measuring cortisol secretion after administration of the glucocorticoid dexamethasone (the dexamethasone suppression test). Cortisol release is suppressed via inhibitory feedback to the hypothalamus mediated by the glucocorticoid receptor. Non-suppression of cortisol occurs in abnormal states such as Cushing's disease and implies either reduced feedback and/or enhanced central drive for its release. The dexamethasone suppression test was shown to have a high specificity and sensitivity for severe depression compared with control patients in early studies but it is less useful for discriminating between different patient groups. There appears to be hypertrophy of the adrenal glands in major depression, with a measurable increase in size on MRI, and an enhanced response to a fixed dose of corticotropin. Like the hypercortisolemia, the MRI change is reversible on recovery. However, relatively impaired glucocorticoid feedback has also been described in relatives of depressed patients who do not have mood disorder and in euthymic bipolar patients.

Early experiences of stress influence steroid responses in adult animals, and so the HPA axis provides a potential link between adverse early experience and subsequent mood disorder. In the case of bipolar disorder, such early experience does not appear to cause adult illness but it does appear to make the outcomes worse.

It is unclear whether endogenous cortisol actually contributes to the clinical picture of depression and mania by a direct action on the brain; if it does, it may mediate at least part of the postulated stress-diathesis model in mood disorder. Administration of cortisol is certainly associated with affective symptoms. Acute dosing can precipitate euphoria and, in bipolar I patients, the full syndrome of mania. Long-term treatment or excessive chronic cortisol secretion can produce depressive symptoms, as in Cushing's disease. If 'cortisol toxicity' does indeed contribute to mood disorders, antagonism of the actions of cortisol could have important psychotropic effects; convincing evidence is awaited.

Although steroids are measured in the extracellular compartment, the primary actions are currently understood to be on intracellular receptors. It is striking that the hypercortisolemia of mood disorder is not associated with the metabolic changes seen in Cushing's disease. This is puzzling, unless the transport of steroids across the plasma membrane is disturbed in mood disorder. From this hypothesis follows an interesting new idea that high extracellular levels of cortisol could coexist or even be provoked by low local intracellular levels of cortisol.

### Other endocrine abnormalities

**Thyroid dysfunction.** Hyperthyroidism is characterized by increased anxiety and emotional lability; it may even present as hypomania or mania. Hypothyroidism is classically associated with a reversible dementia, although depressive features may also be prominent. As thyroid dysfunction commonly disrupts the psyche, does psychiatric disorder have reciprocal associations with thyroid dysfunction? Abnormalities of the thyroid axis in bipolar disorder have often been described. Unfortunately, however, there is a particular confounding factor – the use of lithium. Lithium interferes with the peripheral action of thyrotropin in the thyroid, and tends to raise thyrotropin and lower thyroid hormone levels in the blood. Nevertheless, mild hypothyroidism appears to be associated with rapid cycling, and the thyrotropin response to thyrotropin-releasing hormone is blunted in some patients with depression. Furthermore, thyroid hormones have been used in the treatment of rapid cycling and refractory depression. There is also evidence that thyroxine has important interactions with neurotransmitter systems within the brain; if these are abnormally regulated in mood disorder – norepinephrine may be a particular candidate – then the basis for these often neglected clinical associations may prove extremely interesting.

**Insulin abnormalities.** Elevation in insulin levels and vulnerability to insulin resistance has also been associated with bipolar disorder. This may account for the increased rates of obesity, type 2 diabetes and polycystic ovarian syndrome that have been reported in bipolar patients. The extent to which vulnerability to insulin resistance is a risk factor for bipolar disorder, a consequence of treatments or a reflection of lifestyle choices remains to be clarified.

## Biological rhythms and sleep disturbance

The seasonality and cyclicity of bipolar disorder suggests that the sleep–wake cycle may play a fundamental role in the pathophysiology. Patients with severe depression may respond to sleep deprivation with a transient increase in mood. Sleep disturbance is associated with, and may contribute to, processes that initiate the onset of mania. It remains a reasonable hypothesis that sleep disturbance is a final common pathway through which a variety of stressors may operate to trigger mood episodes in patients with bipolar I disorder.

## Functional neuropathology

The neuropathology of brain diseases is often characterized by the appearance of abnormal proteins. These can provide the first molecular signature of the disorder, such as the plaques and tangles in Alzheimer's disease. Psychiatric disorders do not generally have a pathology detectable on gross inspection or under light microscopy. This has led to the designation of psychiatric disorder, perhaps tastelessly, as a graveyard for pathologists. Some objections to a medical approach to psychiatry also rest on this apparent failure.

Methods for quantifying cell number and synaptic connectivity have improved in recent years, leading to the discovery that certain areas of the limbic cortex are in fact abnormal in patients with mood disorder. The reduction in cell numbers appears to be most striking in the glial cell population, but the associated changes in synaptic density obviously involve neurons. Although the abnormality is quantitative rather than qualitative, it could constitute the basis for the subtle but pervasive symptoms of mood disorder and may explain the tendency for recurrence. Caution is still required because there may be alternative explanations. However, a functional or even synaptic neuropathology is a plausible unifying explanation for much of what is seen clinically.

## Neuroimaging

Neuroimaging has revealed little that is practically helpful for the diagnosis, management and treatment of bipolar disorder. However, as already indicated, imaging has transformed cognitive neuroscience and our approach to psychopathology in the past decade. As techniques are refined, imaging is likely to contribute much more to our understanding of abnormal structure and connectivity in the brains of individual patients with bipolar disorder. The key hypothesis is that neural networks that regulate emotional processing in the brain are somehow vulnerable to acute decompensation – the episodes we see as clinicians. This vulnerability is likely to be expressed in abnormal connectivity, which is potentially detectable in individuals using sensitive methods such as diffusion tensor imaging, positron emission tomography or spectroscopy. Moreover, repeated episodes of illness may themselves cause additional damage to these networks and make their further disruption more detectable by imaging methods. Preliminary evidence is now emerging that gray matter density is indeed serially impaired by recurrent episodes. Today, the prospects for real conceptual and practical advances are more exciting than they have been for many years.

## Key points – etiology

- Bipolar I disorder is a highly heritable condition. The present evidence suggests a contribution from multiple genes of modest or small effect.
- Unlike schizophrenia, there is little evidence for an environmental factor or a neurodevelopmental defect.
- Family studies show an excess of unipolar depression and psychosis among bipolar patients, suggesting that the polygenic inheritance is expressed as a variety of related phenotypes.
- The genes so far implicated appear to be of small effect; they appear to control brain development rather than ongoing neurotransmission.
- Current genetic findings do not support a role for clinical genetic testing for bipolar disorder.
- Dopamine hyperactivity appears to be directly implicated in the neurobiology of manic symptoms.
- Bipolar depression, unlike unipolar forms, may not be securely linked to decreased function of serotonin. Norepinephrine may be implicated in bipolar depression and there may be enduring deficits in sustained attention in euthymic bipolar patients.
- Cortisol and thyroid hormones have been implicated in mood disorder. An acute excess of either tends to produce euphoria. Long-term hypercortisolemia may produce depression. Abnormalities of the hypothalamic–pituitary–adrenal and thyroid axes are often described in euthymic bipolar patients.
- Sleep is similarly disrupted in mania and depression. A direct euphoriant effect of sleep deprivation may be relevant to the evolution of the manic state.

## Key references

Arts B, Jabben N, Krabbendam L, van Os J. Meta-analyses of cognitive functioning in euthymic bipolar patients and their first-degree relatives. *Psychol Med* 2008;38: 771–85.

Braff DL, Freedman R. Clinically responsible genetic testing in neuropsychiatric patients: a bridge too far and too soon. *Am J Psychiatry* 2008;165:952–5.

Craddock N, O'Donovan MC, Owen MJ. Genome-wide association studies in psychiatry: lessons from early studies of non-psychiatric and psychiatric phenotypes. *Mol Psychiatry* 2008;13:649–53.

Cummings JL, Mendez MF. Secondary mania with focal cerebrovascular lesions. *Am J Psychiatry* 1984;141:1084–7.

Gershon ES, Hamovit J, Guroff JJ et al. A family study of schizoaffective, bipolar I, bipolar II, unipolar, and normal control probands. *Arch Gen Psychiatry* 1982;39:1157–67.

Goodwin FK, Jamison KR. *Manic-Depressive Illness: Bipolar Disorders and Recurrent Depression*, 2nd edn. Oxford: Oxford University Press, 2007.

Harrison PJ. The neuropathology of primary mood disorder. *Brain* 2002;125:1428–49.

McTavish SF, Mcpherson MH, Harmer CJ et al. Antidopaminergic effects of dietary tyrosine depletion in healthy subjects and patients with manic illness. *Br J Psychiatry* 2001; 179:356–60.

Moorhead TW, McKirdy J, Sussmann JE et al. Progressive gray matter loss in patients with bipolar disorder. *Biol Psychiatry* 2007;62: 894–900.

Sklar P, Smoller JW, Fan J et al. Whole-genome association study of bipolar disorder. *Mol Psychiatry* 2008;13:558–69.

Tsai SY, Lee HC, Chen CC. Hyperinsulinaemia associated with beta-adrenoceptor antagonist in medicated bipolar patients during manic episode. *Prog Neuropsychopharmacol Biol Psychiatry* 2007;31:1038–43.

Tsankova N, Renthal W, Kumar A, Nestler EJ. Epigenetic regulation in psychiatric disorders. *Nat Rev Neurosci* 2007;8:355–67.

Videbech P. MRI findings in patients with affective disorder: a meta-analysis. *Acta Psychiatr Scand* 1997;96:157–68.

Wehr TA, Sack DA, Rosenthal NE. Sleep reduction as a final common pathway in the genesis of mania. *Am J Psychiatry* 1987;144:201–4.

Bipolar I disorder, defined by the occurrence of mania and usually diagnosed during hospital admission for mania, is a relatively rare condition with a lifetime incidence of approximately 1% in the general population. The lifetime incidence of bipolar II disorder diagnosed using DSM-IV criteria is also about 1%, and bipolar disorder not otherwise specified (NOS) contributes a further 2.4%. The total is equivalent to more than 5 million US adults and 1 million in the UK. Again using DSM-IV criteria, unipolar depression is by far the commonest mood disorder in the community, affecting 16% of the National Comorbidity Replication Sample in the USA and 21% of the Zurich sample shown on the left-hand side of Figure 3.1.

The diagnosis of bipolar II disorder remains controversial because of the boundary of hypomania with normality, rather than its boundary with mania. The issue is deceptively simple: how to draw the line between a patient who has experienced episodes of elation and one who has not.

It turns out that many people experience and describe short-term changes in mood that fail to meet the DSM-IV criteria for hypomania. However, the phenomenon is often associated with other morbidity (e.g. depression, deliberate self-harm and substance misuse) and, on this basis, Angst has argued for a more liberal definition of hypomania. The more liberal the definition, the more inclusive it becomes, bringing cases of major depression into what is often called the 'bipolar spectrum'. This expansion of the concept of hypomania inflates the bipolar diagnosis shown in Figure 3.1.

The clinical message, already emphasized in Chapter 1, is a relatively straightforward one. In addition to diagnosing depression in patients presenting to primary care physicians, or indeed to psychiatrists, inquiries should also be made about periods of excessive energy, decreased need for sleep, heightened sexual interest, increased risk taking, enhanced cognitive ability and elation. At present, a positive response to such inquiries and a provisional diagnosis of bipolar spectrum disorder is not

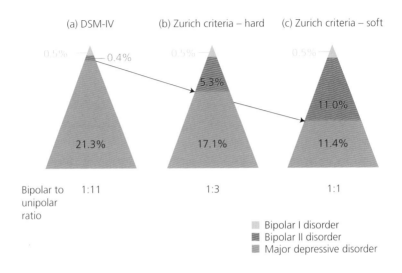

**Figure 3.1** The lifetime incidence of bipolar disorder depends on how bipolar II disorder is defined. (a) Applying DSM-IV criteria, the lifetime incidence of bipolar I and II disorder together is about 1%. Unipolar major depressive disorder is much more common under this definition. If the diagnosis of bipolar II disorder is liberalized, the number of patients with major depressive disorder who are reclassified as having bipolar II disorder will expand. (b) and (c) show expansion of the percentage of bipolar II patients for successively more inclusive definitions using the Zurich criteria. The hard criteria imply behavioral consequences of hypomanic mood disturbance, while the soft criteria do not. Data and Zurich criteria from Angst J et al., 2003.

a clear indication for action. It is, however, an indication for caution, particularly in the use of antidepressants (see below).

## Burden of disease

Mood disorders are among the leading causes of morbidity and mortality in western and developing countries. This can obviously be seen primarily as an accumulation of personal misery. Mood disorders cause disability because they impair cognition and prevent people from working for long periods of time. This causes absenteeism, which is obvious, but patients with depression who return to work may be ineffective and contribute to a problem often called presenteeism. The combined impact of depression in the world of work is very large and is now attracting the interest of major employers. Bipolar cases contribute disproportionately to this toll.

Morbidity is particularly high because the age of onset is usually young. How young remains controversial and merits a full discussion.

## Children and young adults

The incidence of bipolar disorder is a function of age. Although a first episode of mania may be seen in patients over 80 years old, the peak decade is 15–25 years. Anyone who has spent up to 6 months working in an acute psychiatric unit will have seen a young person admitted to hospital in a wildly excited manic state, much to the consternation of friends and family. This is the traditional view of how bipolar disorder starts.

There is now an alternative view that much earlier diagnosis should be possible if more sensitive instruments are used and a broadly conceived phenotype is accepted that recognizes chronic mixed features, particularly irritability, as the predominant expression of prepubertal bipolar disorder. This perspective largely grows out of the experience of psychiatrists working with children and adolescents in the USA. On this basis, the diagnosis of bipolar disorder in quite young children is becoming increasingly common – and controversial. It represents another of the ways in which practice in North America is different from that in most other parts of the world; a parallel trend has not yet been described in other countries, where bipolar disorder is almost never diagnosed before the age of 10 years.

There are at least two different ways to interpret this difference. First, there may indeed be developmental abnormalities in children who are later diagnosed as having bipolar disorder and these may be expressed as identifiable mood-congruent behavioral changes. With careful rating and attention to clinical detail, the diagnosis is now being claimed in children as young as 5 years. However, the instruments on which these claims rely are essentially modifications of adult rating scales to reflect what are interpreted as 'manic' features in children. There is an explicit softening of the edges of diagnostic criteria in an effort to detect a juvenile equivalent of the signal psychopathology seen in adults with bipolar disorder. Whether this is a valid procedure can be determined only on the basis of its predictive power: how many children detected in this way actually develop conventionally defined bipolar disorder, and – just as importantly – how many do not. It is still possible for the skeptic to say that this is diagnosis inflation; the more pessimistic would argue that it may be leading to the misdiagnosis (and mistreatment) of more children than it actually satisfactorily identifies.

The second approach is to take the data at face value and propose that something is happening in the USA to make bipolar symptoms more common in children. One possible explanation is the widespread use of stimulants for the treatment of hyperactivity. Figures vary, but as many as 10% of some school populations receive stimulants for this indication and, as hyperactivity could be a precursor of bipolar disorder, it is possible that exposure to amphetamine-like agents may precipitate earlier appearance of bipolar disorder than would otherwise have occurred. Some data from US clinics support this. Other possibilities include nutritional and cultural factors, which may accelerate the trend of expression of mood disorder at a younger age.

This situation presents a dilemma to the clinician. Parents may be keen for their children to be diagnosed with bipolar disorder early so that they can receive effective treatment. However, as we attempt to diagnose positively on the basis of predictive psychopathology, we will be less reliable and more prone to initiate treatment inappropriately. We believe this dilemma can best be managed by following an approach that relies on formal diagnostic assessment techniques as opposed to rating scales or screening tools. It also requires a narrow rather than a broad definition of mood elevation in children before puberty. In other words, a diagnosis of mania must recognize grandiosity rather than just irritability, which is too common in children to be a reliable indicator of mania. Moreover, a manic state must be episodic not chronic. These simple restrictions provide a firm grounding for a bipolar diagnosis, as studies show that children and adolescents meeting these criteria tend to have a course of illness like that of adult bipolar illness. Investigation and treatment studies of early-onset bipolar disorder are badly needed to guide practice in this area.

In adolescence, the diagnosis of bipolar I disorder from an episode meeting the full criteria for mania becomes increasingly reliable. But, in an attempt to understand the disorder, parents and family members may look back to earlier problems, presume they were part of the illness, and complain that the diagnosis was missed. Such non-specific difficulties should not be indiscriminately linked with the specific development of bipolar disorder, because to do so places a burden on clinicians that even those using the most rigorous research techniques would be ill-equipped to bear.

It will be clear that this review comes at a watershed for early diagnosis. Clinicians and patients must hope that definitive results

---

**Key points – epidemiology**

- The lifetime incidence of bipolar I disorder is approximately 1%. The lifetime incidence of conservatively defined DSM-IV bipolar II disorder is also about 1%. DSM-IV bipolar NOS (not otherwise specified) is found in a further 2.4%.
- A more liberal diagnosis of hypomania will lead to a higher incidence of bipolar disorder that will include many cases now diagnosed as 'unipolar' major depression.
- Clinicians should inquire about a personal and family history of mood elevation when making a diagnosis of depression.
- Even when defined conservatively, bipolar disorder imposes a major worldwide burden of disease.
- The diagnosis of bipolar disorder in children is controversial. The incidence described in North America is much higher than in the rest of the world, where it is rarely diagnosed before the age of 10 years.
- Diagnostic confidence is increased in subsets of children and adolescents demonstrating discrete episodes with grandiosity/euphoria rather than chronic mood instability with irritability.
- Screening instruments and symptom severity scales are not a substitute for a formal clinical diagnostic assessment.

emerge in the next few years. This is an area that demands patience and caution because it is potentially highly controversial. If we make diagnoses of bipolar disorder in very young children, we may be able to treat them by extrapolating from adult experience. We may even produce a better long-term outcome than would otherwise have been possible. However, there are competing risks. If we use modified criteria to make the diagnosis, how reliable can we expect it to be? How many children do we treat 'unnecessarily' as a consequence? How good are the data to ensure that the medical approaches we extrapolate from adults are either safe or effective in children? Medical practice often involves making unpalatable choices. This area is no exception.

### Key references

Akiskal HS, Bourgeois ML, Angst J et al. Re-evaluating the prevalence of and diagnostic composition within the broad clinical spectrum of bipolar disorders. *J Affect Disord* 2000; 59(suppl 1):S5–30.

Angst J. The emerging epidemiology of hypomania and bipolar II disorder. *J Affect Disord* 1998;50:143–51.

Angst J, Gamma A, Benazzi F et al. Toward a re-definition of subthreshold bipolarity: epidemiology and proposed criteria for bipolar-II, minor bipolar disorders and hypomania. *J Affect Disord* 2003;73:133–46.

Geller B, Tillman R, Craney JL, Bolhofner K. Four-year prospective outcome and natural history of mania in children with a prepubertal and early adolescent bipolar disorder phenotype. *Arch Gen Psychiatry* 2004;61:459–67.

Harrington R, Myatt T. Is preadolescent mania the same condition as adult mania? A British perspective. *Biol Psychiatry* 2003; 53:961–9.

Harris EC, Barraclough B. Suicide as an outcome for mental disorders. A meta-analysis. *Br J Psychiatry* 1997; 170:205–28.

Judd LL, Akiskal HS, Schettler PJ et al. The long-term natural history of the weekly symptomatic status of bipolar I disorder. *Arch Gen Psychiatry* 2002;59:530–7.

Kessler RC, Merikangas KR, Wang PS. Prevalence, comorbidity, and service utilization for mood disorders in the United States at the beginning of the twenty-first century. *Annu Rev Clin Psychol* 2007;3: 137–58.

Murray CJL, Lopez AD. Alternative projections of mortality and disability by cause 1990–2020: Global Burden of Disease Study. *Lancet* 1997;349:1498–504.

Murray CJL, Lopez AD. Global mortality, disability, and the contribution of risk factors: Global Burden of Disease Study. *Lancet* 1997;349:1436–42.

ten Have M, Vollebergh W, Bijl R, Nolen WA. Bipolar disorder in the general population in the Netherlands (prevalence, consequences and care utilisation): results from The Netherlands Mental Health Survey and Incidence Study (NEMESIS). *J Affect Disord* 2002;68:203–13.

Youngstrom EA, Birmaher B, Findling RL. Pediatric bipolar disorder: validity, phenomenology, and recommendations for diagnosis. *Bipolar Disord* 2008;10:194–214.

A consistent and distressing observation frequently made by patients with mood disorder is that their problems and suffering are not taken seriously. This is not just a failing of doctors – it extends to most people they encounter.

Depression, in a variety of forms, from the mild and nagging dysphoria that may last for months to the paralyzing grips of suicidal despair, is a condition that few who have not suffered it can truly claim to understand. Reality seems different after such experiences. By contrast, the euphoria and excitement of mania, the seemingly endless possibilities, the blinding insights and the excitement of feeling powerful, active and hypersexual are experiences that may be highly valued and difficult to relinquish.

The facts given in the preceding chapters largely omit such rich personal experience in favor of a starvation diet of symptoms, diagnoses and frequencies of occurrence. Although this approach may appear to be a further denial of the patient's reality, this is not the case, and in fact the scientific approach is vital.

## Scientific psychiatry

Clinicians do not wish to diminish the value of individual experience; nor do they necessarily fail to understand and sympathize (although this may happen, of course). Accomplished clinicians seek what is common in form or content in the stories patients tell them, not what is unique.

There is good reason for this scientific approach to psychiatric disorders: it offers reliable knowledge, not anecdote. Indeed, all that science is, ultimately, is reliable knowledge. And it is often just such knowledge that patients seek from their doctors about their illness – how long it will last, whether it will recur, whether it runs in families and what the best treatment is.

Doctors may be wise to make neither friends of their patients nor patients of their friends. This traditional slogan of safe practice places the science of medicine on a different basis from the content of everyday human contact.

Scientific knowledge is reliable because it is reductionist. Mania is defined by reference to a checklist of symptoms – we then know what anyone using the term in a technical way actually means. It is also possible to estimate the probability of mania developing in a lifetime, and the prevalence in a population and in a service. We can then start to generate hypotheses about the underlying cause (e.g. whether or not it is genetic) and conduct trials that measure outcomes with different treatments. Investigators tend to prefer outcomes that are also clearly defined and narrow – seeming to leave out what 'matters most' to an individual in favor of what we think captures measurable, but meaningful, change in the clinical state. This approach is underpinned by the principle that if an approach is wrong, then it will be found out by our inability to replicate results and failure to move on to more fruitful hypotheses. Scientific ideas are falsifiable; anecdote and personal experience are not, and have to be judged by other quasi-literary standards.

Reliable knowledge about any natural phenomenon increases as more effort is put into research. In the past, every severe illness was a mysterious personal journey to death or disability to which almost any mythology could be attached. Over the last century, medicine has generally been transformed by just such a scientific approach to the definition of illness, investigation and treatment in every specialty. Arguably, psychiatry has been the slowest specialty to adopt science wholeheartedly and it also happens to deal with the subtlest disturbances of personal function – in emotion, thinking and behavior. However, psychiatric illnesses are responsible for the deaths of millions of people every year through suicide, and rank as leading causes of disability worldwide. If such disorders could be better treated, fewer people would die, or suffer, unnecessarily. That, in essence, is why doctors hold the views that we do and try to make our practice more scientific.

Science also provides the basis for what we want all patients to know about their illness. That knowledge may be crucial to their self-management and to the effective contribution of family and friends. It not only includes the effective use of medicines and the need for adherence to what is prescribed, though that is very important, but also understanding why lifestyle changes may be necessary and how specific psychological treatments may provide benefit. These are key factors in enhancement of care.

## Patients' experiences

A scientific acceptance of the facts of bipolar disorder, and how to treat it, presents no barrier to listening to the life stories of bipolar patients. The compelling human interest these narratives often provoke may reflect their extreme expression of the triumphs, tragedies and striving of our common humanity. Indeed, there appears to be a fundamental connection between mood disorder and artistic or literary creativity. Kay Jamison's masterly survey *Touched with Fire* makes an overwhelming case. Some of the greatest artists who have ever lived provide a treasure trove of their experience of mood disorder. The following descriptions give a brief impression of what the experience may be like.

Of mania, Kay Jamison wrote in *An Unquiet Mind*:

> *Even now I can see in my mind's rather peculiar eye an extraordinary shattering and shifting of light; inconstant but ravishing colours laid out across miles of circling rings; and the almost imperceptible, somehow surprisingly pallid moons of this Catherine wheel of a planet. I remember singing 'Fly me to the moons' as I swept past those of Saturn ... Long after my psychosis cleared ... it became part of what one remembers forever.*

> (Jamison KR. *An Unquiet Mind. A Memoir of Moods and Madness.*)

However, mania is a transient state; more stable hyperthymic traits are associated with bipolar disorder. Nigel Nicholson described Virginia Woolf's conversation thus:

> *One would hand her a bit of information, as dull as a lump of lead, and she would hand it back glittering with diamonds. I always felt on leaving that I had drunk two glasses of excellent champagne. Virginia was a life enhancer.*

> (Caramagno T. *The Flight of the Mind.*)

Hyperthymia and even hypomania probably provide the key to the high achievement of creative people with bipolar disorder.

The famous writers, poets, composers and artists listed in Table 4.1 almost certainly experienced severe mood disorder. Depression is the most pervasive consequence of bipolar disorder, and the best documented clinical state in these individuals. However, many clearly experienced mania, and showed bursts of productivity likely related to hypomania.

As we have already seen, alcohol and drug misuse are common comorbidities of bipolar disorder, and personal difficulties of all sorts may be aggravated by abnormal moods. Accordingly, many of those listed in Table 4.1 are better known for substance misuse and/or the chaos of their private lives than for the mood disorder that will often have played a causal part.

In less articulate forms, such material is also present in every outpatient clinic in which individuals with bipolar disorder are seen and, more importantly, heard.

That some of the very best poetry, literature and visual art are wrought by writers and artists from the experience of mood disorder is extraordinary. Why then is the salience in artists' lives of such illnesses so poorly appreciated by the general and even the literary public? There are at least two important explanations.

First, the extremes of experience that torture artists in the psychotic extremes of mania or depression do not usually provide the literal fabric for their work, however much they may indirectly inform it. Indeed, there is an exceedingly important distinction between madness and creativity.

The creative thrust of psychosis tends, like that of drug intoxication, to be hollow and pointless unless there is a euthymic censor to create the work of art – creativity needs control, restraint, editorial structure. A writer's illness may be effectively edited from their work, unless one is sufficiently sensitive to find it. The work of Robert Lowell, arguably the most important US poet of the last century, can be used to illustrate this point. The poem shown on page 49 does not refer to mood, but its fluency and richness of association shows it may originate in hypomania.

TABLE 4.1

**Famous creative artists who almost certainly experienced severe mood disorder**

Writers

- Hans Christian Andersen
- Honoré de Balzac
- Samuel Clemens (Mark Twain)
- Joseph Conrad (SA)
- Charles Dickens
- Ralph Waldo Emerson
- William Faulkner (H)
- F Scott Fitzgerald (H)
- Lewis Grassic Gibbon (SA)
- Maxim Gorky (SA)
- Kenneth Graham
- Graham Greene
- Ernest Hemingway (H, S)
- Hermann Hesse (H, SA)
- Henrik Ibsen
- Henry James
- Charles Lamb (H)
- Malcolm Lowry (H, S)
- Herman Melville
- Eugene O'Neill (H, SA)
- John Ruskin (H)
- Mary Shelley
- Robert Louis Stevenson
- August Strindberg
- Leo Tolstoy
- Ivan Turgenev
- Tennessee Williams (H)
- Mary Wollstonecraft (SA)
- Virginia Woolf (H, S)

Poets

- Antonin Artaud (H)
- Charles Baudelaire (SA)
- Thomas Lovell Beddoes (S)
- John Berryman (H, S)
- William Blake
- Robert Burns
- George Gordon, Lord Byron
- Thomas Chatterton (S)
- John Clare (H)
- Samuel Taylor Coleridge
- William Cowper (H, SA)
- Hart Crane (S)
- John Davidson (S)
- Emily Dickinson
- TS Eliot (H)
- Sergei Esenin (S)
- Robert Fergusson (H)
- Oliver Goldsmith
- Thomas Gray
- Friedrich Hölderlin (H)
- Gerard Manley Hopkins
- Victor Hugo
- Randal Jarrell (H, S)
- Samuel Johnson
- John Keats
- Heinrich Von Kleist (S)
- Vachel Lindsay (S)
- Robert Lowell (H)
- Hugh MacDiarmid (H)
- Louis MacNeice
- Osip Mandelstam (H, SA)
- Vladimir Mayakovsky (S)
- Gerard de Nerval (H, S)

CONTINUED

TABLE 4.1 (CONTINUED)

- Boris Pasternak (H)
- Cesare Pavese (S)
- Sylvia Plath (H, S)
- Edgar Allan Poe (SA)
- Ezra Pound (H)
- Alexander Pushkin
- Laura Riding (SA)
- Theodore Roethke (H)
- Delmore Schwartz (H)
- Anne Sexton (H, S)
- Percy Bysshe Shelley (SA)
- Torquato Tasso (H)
- Alfred, Lord Tennyson
- Dylan Thomas
- George Trakl (H, S)
- Marina Tsvetayeva (S)
- Walt Whitman

Composers

- Hector Berlioz (SA)
- Anton Bruckner (H)
- Jeremiah Clarke (S)
- John Dowland
- Edward Elgar
- Mikhail Glinka
- George Frederic Handel
- Gustav Holst
- Charles Ives
- Otto Klemperer (H)
- Orlando de Lassus
- Gustav Mahler
- Modest Mussorgsky
- Sergey Rachmaninoff
- Giocchino Rossini
- Robert Schumann (H, S)

- Alexander Scriabin
- Peter Tchaikovsky
- Peter Warlock (S)
- Hugo Wolf (H, SA)
- Bernd Alois Zimmerman (S)

Artists

- Ralph Barton (S)
- Francesco Bassano (S)
- Francesco Borromini (S)
- Richard Dadd (H)
- Edward Dayes (S)
- Paul Gauguin (SA)
- Théodore Géricault
- Hugo van der Goes
- Vincent van Gogh (H, S)
- Arshile Gorky (S)
- Philip Guston (H)
- Benjamin Haydon (S)
- George Innes (SA)
- Ernst Josephson (H)
- Ernst Ludwig Kirchner (H, S)
- Edwin Landseer (H)
- Edward Lear
- Michelangelo Buonarroti
- Edvard Munch (H)
- Georgia O'Keeffe (H)
- Jules Pascin (S)
- Jackson Pollock (H)
- Dante Gabriel Rossetti (SA)
- Mark Rothko (S)
- Nicolas de Staël (S)
- Henry Tilson (S)
- Sir David Wilkie

H, admitted at least once to an asylum or psychiatric hospital; S, suicide; SA, suicide attempt.
Adapted with permission from Kay Redfield Jamison. *Touched with Fire: Manic-Depressive Illness and the Artistic Temperament.* New York: Free Press, 1993.

Second, psychiatric illness is stigmatizing. It takes courage to talk about these disorders, and this may be particularly true in a literary milieu, where there may be a good deal of denial that such illness is real, or there may be a vindictive desire to explain why it has happened in terms of the sufferer's personal relationships. Literary biography is often littered with fanciful explanation of why things turned out as they did, and is at its weakest when explaining away psychiatric illness. Sylvia Plath's husband, Ted Hughes, was subjected to remarkable criticism that implied he was responsible for her death by suicide, even though her diaries and her work show that her debilitating depressive states were recurrent from a time before they had met.

In our view, the failure to embrace and understand scientific accounts of mood disorder promotes stigma and superstition. We need reliable accounts of the world. Understanding that the Earth goes round the Sun does not make the sunrise less beautiful, but it does make it less likely that human sacrifices will be made to ensure it goes on happening.

## Terminology and stigma

To reduce the stigma of mood disorders in general, and bipolar disorder in particular, champions are needed who can emerge from the closet and talk about what it is like to be affected. Because so many talented people have suffered from bipolar disorder, we do now have a literature of this sort.

William Styron has written rivetingly about the experience of depression and here reflects on how we use and understand language:

> *Depression ... used to be termed melancholia ... 'Melancholia' would still appear to be a far more apt and evocative word for the blacker forms of the disorder, but it was usurped by a noun with a bland tonality and lacking any magisterial presence, used indifferently to describe an economic decline or a rut in the ground, a true wimp of a word.*
>
> (Styron W. Darkness Visible. *A Memoir of Madness*.)

We certainly need to be alert to the nuances of terminology that do not ring true to patients; for example, the term 'bipolar' is

EPILOGUE
## Robert Lowell (1917–77)

Those blessèd structures, plot and rhyme –
why are they no help to me now
I want to make
something imagined, not recalled?
I hear the noise of my own voice:
The painter's vision is not a lens, it trembles to caress the light.
But sometimes everything I write
with the threadbare art of my eye
seems a snapshot,
lurid, rapid, garish, grouped,
heightened from life,
yet paralyzed by fact.
All's misalliance.
Yet why not say what happened?
Pray for the grace of accuracy
Vermeer gave to the sun's illumination
stealing like the tide across a map
to his girl solid with yearning.
We are poor passing facts,
warned by that to give
each figure in the photograph
his living name.

Reproduced with permission from Bidart R, Gewanter D, eds. *The Collected Poems of Robert Lowell.* London: Faber & Faber, 2003.

preferred to 'manic-depressive' by many patients and is now used much more widely.

It is questionable whether we should give in to more politicized attempts to change terminology. Such changes appear to arise from more totalitarian motives. A particular example is the very term 'patient'. We use the term patient because we find it to be widely understood and it places psychiatric patients on equal terms with patients with other diseases. Its original meaning – a sufferer – made it a

49

natural choice to describe those under medical care, at least for the last 600 years or so. The currently competing words are interesting.

- Client (from the Latin, originally describing the dependent relationship of a plebian to a patrician) is often deliberately used by psychologists and nurses to distinguish their relationship with patients from that of doctors. Quite how it incorporates a difference in practice or 'model', which is often implied, is not widely understood or, perhaps, understandable. The other connotations of the term client can be less satisfactory, conjuring up images of lawyers or prostitutes.
- The word consumer is more neutral, but implies a degree of choice many patients do not enjoy.
- The term user (of services) or service user is widely promoted, and even imposed, by current Department of Health policy in the UK. It reflects dissatisfaction with all references to illness or illness connotations in 'mental health' services. Whether this denial of why we need such services at all will prove to be more or less stigmatizing is a moot point. If it proves inimical to a scientific approach to psychiatry, it will be a disaster.

We accept the key issue that clinicians must respect their patients as people who happen to have a mood disorder and never as diagnoses with an almost irrelevant human being attached. Good clinicians will hear their patients' stories and will understand some, at least, of the personal meanings these stories have, but they should not be seduced into thinking that this is ever enough. The best thing a doctor can do for his or her patient is to weigh the salience and reliability of information from history and examination in order to formulate an accurate diagnosis and offer appropriate treatment. This, together with a constructive therapeutic alliance, are essential elements in what we regard as the enhancement of care.

## Key points – the patient's perspective

- Mood disorder imposes extreme experiences on patients and their families, which are poorly appreciated by the general public and, too often perhaps, by clinicians.
- Mood disorder has played a central part in the lives of a disproportionate number of creative artists. Hypomania may lie at the core of extreme bursts of creative energy. Mania and depression contribute crucial experiences to the lives of creative artists, but madness is not the same as creativity.
- The relationship between mood disorder and creative experience is an important one, but states of frank mania or depression are rarely compatible with effective thought or action.
- The patient's personal story is important to understanding the context and meaning of any illness.
- The scientific approach to diagnosis and treatment, which we unreservedly favor, is fully compatible with a humane and compassionate relationship with the patient.

### Key references

Caramagno T. *The Flight of the Mind*. Berkeley: University of California Press, 1992. (A detailed account of Virginia Woolf's bipolar disorder.)

Jamison KR. *Touched with Fire: Manic-Depressive Illness and the Artistic Temperament*. New York and London: Simon & Schuster, 1994.

Jamison KR. *An Unquiet Mind. A Memoir of Moods and Madness*. London: Picador, 1996.

Lish JD, Dime-Meenan S, Whybrow PC et al. The National Depressive and Manic-Depressive Association (DMDA) survey of bipolar members. *J Affect Disord* 1994;31:281–94.

Lowell R. In: Bidart F, Gewanter D, eds. *The Collected Poems of Robert Lowell*. London: Faber & Faber, 2003.

Perlick D, Clarkin JF, Sirey J et al. Burden experienced by care-givers of persons with bipolar affective disorder. *Br J Psychiatry* 1999;175:56–62.

Styron W. *Darkness Visible. A Memoir of Madness*. New York: Random House, 1990.

Woolf V. *Mrs Dalloway*. Orlando: Harcourt, 1990. (First published by Hogarth Press, 1925.)

*"Errors in judgment must occur in the practice of an art which consists largely of balancing probabilities."*

(Osler W. Aequanimitas.)

It makes sense to speak of enhancing care because the care being offered to bipolar patients is currently less than it should be. The basics never change, of course: doctors should take a careful history, conduct a relevant physical examination and make the necessary investigations to formulate their diagnosis. This, and the medical plan of management, should be explained. Communication must be clear and effective. The objective is a therapeutic alliance between doctor and patient, which is essential for the management of a complex chronic condition.

Bipolar patients require more than this, however, because they must assume such a vital self-management role in an illness that can distort perception and judgment. Most succeed only by acquiring knowledge, experience, skill and the ongoing collaboration of friends and relatives.

Clinicians can foster success in this endeavor by using a systematic approach to deliver individualized measurement-based treatment. This approach begins with recognition that bipolar disorder is a chronic condition that will be managed over time with a series of interventions. The long-term goal is to maximize the patient's quality of life by increasing the rate at which patients and clinicians produce wise amicable decisions. The simple schema we offer to achieve this aim (Figure 5.1) requires both clinicians and patients to have a base of knowledge and skills related to bipolar disorder and its management. Their working relationship includes integration of routine measurement into a shared management process.

## Knowledge (or 'psychoeducation')

To formulate treatment options, clinicians need two kinds of knowledge: first, knowledge of pertinent treatment guidelines or the ability to identify proven treatments; second, knowledge of the individual patient.

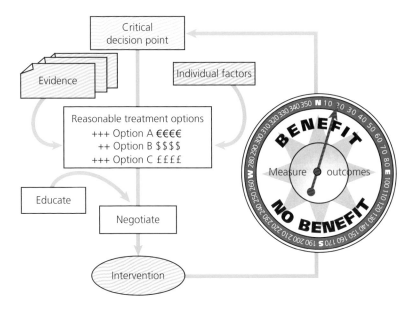

**Figure 5.1** Schema for ongoing measurement-based management.

This includes a broad array of information that might influence choosing a given intervention (e.g. current symptom profile, clinical urgency, previous treatment response, adverse effect tolerance, age, sex, family history).

To maximize the utility of this approach, patients and their supporters are empowered to participate by the provision of basic education about bipolar illness and interventions. Simple negotiation skills can also be taught that foster reaching agreements and maintaining therapeutic alliance (*Getting to Yes* by Fisher et al. is helpful).

Our patients must learn that their acute breakdowns are caused by the chronic illness we call bipolar disorder. Mania and depression in the course of a bipolar illness are not simply understandable responses to stress or one-off problems that are unlikely to recur. Acceptance of these difficult facts is a key early objective of patient education.

Doctors, patients and carers usually start from different positions in building the therapeutic relationship. It is unsurprising that they make different estimates of future risks, as they bring different experiences and beliefs to the process. As already indicated, we believe that patients and

53

carers need to know the facts, as distilled in the preceding chapters of this book. This is essential in order to address the seriousness of the illness, the high risk of relapse and the benefit of active treatment. We cannot expect a patient or carer to know what to do or to do it unless they know why it may make a difference.

Clearly, there is no single way to teach effectively. The efficacy of teaching to a group or class was recently shown in a randomized controlled trial, but we favor a range of didactic teaching approaches, live or by video, written materials or guided Internet searching for high-quality material (see Useful resources on page 107). Educational efforts need to be sustained, and progress is likely to be incremental. A shared and consistent approach across mental health disciplines is helpful, perhaps even essential.

The educational syllabus is effectively the content of this book. Clinicians and other healthcare professionals should not be surprised or feel threatened by patients who appear to know, literally, more than they do. Patients will still need your help when it matters – when they become acutely ill – and they will respect you for not claiming to know everything. Patients, and their supporters as well, will benefit most from education delivered outside periods of acute episodes.

Ultimately, there may be no substitute for experience, however bitter it may be. Doctors must be prepared to understand and eventually harness the repeated triumph of hope over experience that may be required before a patient finally becomes convinced of the need to take self-management seriously. Integration of routine measures can accelerate this process. Much as following blood pressure while patients implement sequential interventions for hypertension aids clinical management, integration of simple routine measures such as global impression ratings, symptom severity scale scores or other standardized notations of clinical status can guide decision-making over the course of bipolar disorder.

## Skills

Once a patient accepts the broad facts about bipolar disorder, they give up a sense of personal responsibility for at least part of what the disorder is about. However, there is a new challenge, which is to identify and adjust the aspects of lifestyle and behavior that may be making things worse. Patients need to acquire skills to manage their mood disorder as effectively as possible.

Patients can learn how to monitor and recognize relevant symptoms or signs and develop an action plan to manage this contingency. For example, sleep disturbance is the most frequently described final common pathway to mania. Shortening of the sleep cycle may be relatively easy to monitor and is susceptible to early treatment by social withdrawal or self-medication. Such early intervention implies patient autonomy. If the focus is sleep disturbance, the patient should keep a benzodiazepine or other hypnotic available. Antipsychotics may also be taken at the onset of a manic episode to reduce its severity. In addition, an increase in the dose of other medicines under specific circumstances may be agreed. This gives the individual a greater sense of control and permits immediate action. It also enables the patient and clinician to evaluate the outcome of various strategies and replace those that are ineffective. Other impulses and preoccupations may form part of the relatively stereotyped prodrome to relapse in individual patients. The involvement of family members may also be helpful, even essential, but must be treated sensitively, as it will not always be welcomed by the patient.

Patients may inadvertently risk relapse by irregular and even reckless patterns of activity and sleep. Establishing routine and regular activity is thus a primary goal of treatment. Daily self-monitoring of mood, anxiety, activity and sleep forms a central component of most enhanced-care packages. Self-monitoring is employed in many psychological treatments and makes good intuitive sense to 40–60% of bipolar patients. Part of a mood chart form is shown in Figure 5.2. (Blank forms with instructions for patients and clinicians can be downloaded from www.manicdepressive.org/tools_all.html)

No treatment plan will work if alcohol or drug misuse is a problem. Abstinence must be an unambiguous treatment goal for such patients.

The general point emerges that outcomes for patients can often be improved by simple commonsense behavioral interventions. Even when ill, it is often possible for patients to get the benefit of the plans made during well states by involving at least one 'care partner' in a written care plan. This trusted carer can help the patient stay on track when the

**MOOD**

Rate with 2 marks each day to indicate best and worst

0 = none
1 = mild
2 = moderate
3 = severe

| Irritability | Anxiety | Hours Slept Last Night | Depressed – Severe: Significant Impairment NOT ABLE TO WORK | Depressed – Mod.: Significant Impairment ABLE TO WORK | Depressed – Mild: Without Significant Impairment | WNL: MOOD NOT DEFINITELY ELEVATED OR DEPRESSED. NO SYMPTOMS. Circle date to indicate Menses | Elevated – Mild: Without Significant Impairment | Elevated – Mod.: Significant Impairment ABLE TO WORK | Elevated – Severe: Significant Impairment NOT ABLE TO WORK | Psychotic Symptoms Strange Ideas, Hallucinations |
|---|---|---|---|---|---|---|---|---|---|---|
| | | | | | | | | | | |
| | | | | | | | | | | |
| | | | | | | | | | | |
| | | | | | | | | | | |
| 2 | 1 | 7 | | | X | X 1 | | | | |
| 2 | 1 | 6 | | X | | 2 X | | | | |
| 2 | 1 | 8 | | X | | X 3 | | | | |
| 1 | 2 | 8 | | | | X 4 | X | | | |
| 1 | 2 | 8 | | | X | X 5 | | | | |
| 1 | 1 | 9 | | X | X | 6 | | | | |
| 1 | 2 | 9 | | X | | X 7 | | | | |
| 1 | 2 | 9 | | X | | X 8 | | | | |
| 1 | 2 | 9 | | X | X | 9 | | | | |
| 1 | 1 | 7 | | X | | 10 X | | | | |
| 1 | 1 | 7 | | | X | 11 X | | | | |
| 1 | 1 | 6 | | | X | X 12 | | | | |
| 1 | 1 | 7 | | X | | X 13 | | | | |
| 1 | 2 | 8 | | | X | X 14 | | | | |
| 2 | 1 | 8 | | | X | X 15 | | | | |
| 1 | 1 | 9 | | | X | X 16 | | | | |
| 1 | 1 | 6 | | | | 17 | X | | | |
| 1 | 1 | 5 | | | X | 18 | | X | | |
| 1 | 1 | 6 | | | | 19 X | | X | | |
| 1 | 1 | 4 | | | | 20 | X | | X | |
| 2 | 2 | 6 | | | | 21 X | | X | | |
| 2 | 2 | 5 | | | | X 22 | | X | | |
| 2 | 2 | 8 | | | X | 23 | | | X | |
| 2 | 2 | 5 | | | | X 24 | | X | | |
| 2 | 2 | 6 | | | | 25 X | | | X | |
| 1 | 3 | 5 | | | | 26 | X | X | | |
| 2 | 2 | 9 | | | | X 27 | | X | | |
| 2 | 3 | 8 | | | X | 28 X | | | | |
| 1 | 2 | 7 | | X | | X 29 | | | | |
| 1 | 2 | 7 | | | X | 30 X | | | | |
| | | | | | | X 31 X | | | | |

**Figure 5.2** Part of a mood chart for a rapid-cycling patient. This illustrates relative mood stability with an excess of depressive symptoms from day 1 to day 16, with a swing from day 17 to more elevated mood and greater instability.

patient's executive function is compromised by illness. Translating this observation into enhanced care for more patients should be an important objective for treatment.

## Family and friends

Community-based services impose appreciable burdens of responsibility and care on the family and friends of patients with bipolar disorder. The perceptions and beliefs that carers hold regarding bipolar disorder, as for other diseases, may have important effects on the burden that is experienced. Perhaps unsurprisingly, accepting an illness model of the problem – rather than blaming the patient – appears to reduce the carer's perception of stress.

## Adherence to medicines

Patient outcomes can be improved by the measures described above for enhancing care, but this approach is not an alternative to long-term treatment with medicines. Moreover, no medicine can work if a patient does not take it. Whether this problem is viewed as non-adherence, poor compliance or a lack of concordance between patient and care provider, it is common across many chronic illnesses and should be addressed as openly and amicably as possible. Bipolar disorder is no exception: up to 50% of patients are non-adherent with treatment. Hence, the response to a course of treatment with inadequate duration or dosage is inconclusive. The progression toward wise decision-making follows from definitive classification of the outcome for each intervention as effective, ineffective or intolerable. Thus, adherence to prescribed medicines is a key issue.

Given the profiles of the existing medicines, it is often assumed that adverse effects are a major reason for early discontinuation. However, data from the UK suggest that only about 15% of non-adherence is attributable to adverse effects (Figure 5.3). The majority of non-adherence appears to occur because patients do not understand the need for treatment or do not want treatment. Reaching agreement (or concordance) with patients on these crucial points as early as possible may be the most salient therapeutic objective in the long-term management of bipolar disorder.

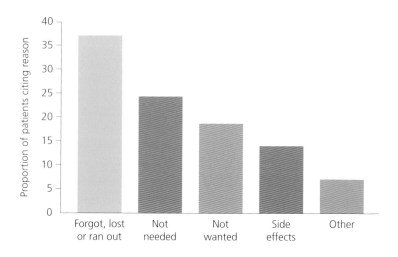

**Figure 5.3** Reasons for non-adherence to medication. Adapted from Cooper et al., 2007.

Management of adverse effects, including those that are subjective (e.g. tiredness and sedation), becomes important in managing those who are concordant with the need for medication. Adverse effects should be minimized by dose adjustments, once-daily administration (e.g. at bedtime) and switching between formulations or comparable medicines. Generic prescribing is more difficult in psychiatry in general, and in mood disorders in particular, because of such complaints. The availability of a formulary that offers a choice between different chemical entities of a similar class is an important and necessary component of enhanced treatment.

Weight gain is a major long-term problem that merits greater prophylactic advice and planning than it usually receives. The monitoring of weight, glucose intolerance and cardiovascular risk factors should be a responsibility that the psychiatrist either undertakes or shares with a primary care physician or specialist.

The motivation to take tablets, particularly in the long term, depends heavily on a knowledge of why the medicines are being prescribed and the balance between cost and benefit perceived by patients and their carers. It is therefore not surprising that psychological interventions can improve adherence and, indeed, that this may account for a large part of the improved outcome associated with psychological approaches (Figure 5.4).

## Cognitive–behavior therapy

Cognitive–behavior therapy (CBT) is widely promoted as an approach to the treatment of mood disorder. It was developed from Beck's specific formulation of a cognitive model for depression. It emphasizes the potential for thoughts and memories to influence mood, rather than vice versa. Its focus is on conscious cognitive biases that may lead patients to make negative interpretations of potentially neutral or even positive events or difficulties. A central ambitious objective is to 'restructure' the patient's negative cognitions.

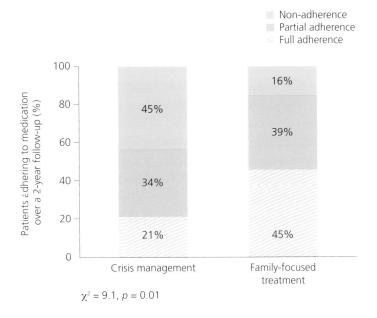

$\chi^2 = 9.1, p = 0.01$

**Figure 5.4** Adherence to prescribed medicines can be improved by high-intensity psychological intervention to increase knowledge, and family communication ('family-focused treatment') when compared with an approach more oriented to crisis management ('crisis management'). Reproduced with permission from Dr D Miklowitz.

In its more refined forms (e.g. in relation to panic disorder), the treatment and its 'mechanism of action' are claimed to be specifically and optimally suited to the psychopathology of the patient's condition. For bipolar disorder, in which a cognitive component is just one of several probable contributing mechanisms, there can be little claim for specificity. CBT is instead a pragmatic approach to the problem that thoughts or beliefs may influence feelings.

When patients are depressed, a variety of psychological interventions may facilitate response. A large effectiveness study in the USA found that adding formal psychosocial interventions (CBT, family-focused therapy and interpersonal social rhythm therapy) to medication for bipolar depression produced a higher rate of response and a more rapid onset of recovery than a control condition.

It has often been assumed that the primary value of CBT would be in preventing relapse. Unfortunately, results of the first major trials of CBT for relapse prevention in bipolar disorder have been conflicting, with the largest discouragingly negative. It is fair to say that generic CBT is unlikely to be the answer for all bipolar patients, particularly those with many previous episodes. More innovation in this area is needed; psychological approaches more specifically tuned to the needs of bipolar patients may well be possible.

Finally, psychotherapy is not always what it purports to be. Regulation is obviously more difficult than for medicines. Some caution may therefore be required when seeking help, especially in the private sector. Patients should not be afraid to ask for proof of professional qualification and evidence of good practice.

### The role of the family

Family-focused therapy has also been formally investigated in adolescents with bipolar disorder and involves their immediate family members (spouse, parents, siblings). It consists of psychoeducation about bipolar disorder, communication enhancement training, and training in problem-solving skills. Overall, it is associated with a worthwhile reduction in recurrence rates over 2 years and a 48% increase in recovery rates over 1 year. Its effects appear to be stronger in stabilizing depressive episodes than in stabilizing manic episodes; it also appears to enhance adherence with lithium and/or anticonvulsant regimens.

## Giving advice: functional impairments

Clinicians will be consulted about expectations and capacity to work. Major decisions should not normally be made by patients in a depressive or manic state. Judgment may be excessively pessimistic in depression, and notoriously optimistic in mania.

Even after recovery from an acute episode, patients may experience unexpected difficulty performing at a level appropriate to their education or training. This may be the consequence of common subsyndromal symptoms of depression or anxiety, or other barriers to psychological well-being. There may even be factors specific to bipolar disorder, such as experience when high, or personality factors, that conspire to widen the gap between aspiration and achievement. Clinical input may be limited to encouragement and appropriate supportive letters, but is often important.

Rather differently, there is now consistent evidence that objective impairments of neuropsychological function are both significant and enduring in patients with bipolar I disorder. These changes appear to be acquired in the wake of recurrent episodes of illness and are evident initially as impairment in sustained attention. More extensive changes in cognitive function extending to memory and executive domains may develop later. Our conviction is that, if these outcomes are avoidable with effective early treatment, then early diagnosis and management will assume increasing importance in the coming years.

Recovery is a sensitive term. For doctors it simply means the return to health and a full range of personal, social and occupational aspirations and achievements. Failure to make a recovery is, by these exacting standards, not uncommon for patients with severe bipolar disorder. There is now a countervailing view – how widely held it is difficult to say – that opposes this and other aspects of the medical model. Instead, recovery is defined against personal goals that may accept a fair level of what might conventionally be described as disability. We can live with both perspectives, but cannot accept that ours is simply wrong.

**Key points – enhanced care**

- Enhancement of patient care is required to improve the capacity of patients to self-manage their bipolar disorder.
- Patients and clinicians require specific knowledge and skills to realize this objective. Successful interventions of all kinds tend to emphasize psychoeducation, self-monitoring and lifestyle modification.
- Abstinence from drugs and alcohol is necessary for effective treatment.
- The adoption of a disciplined and regular pattern of everyday activity is believed to facilitate mood stability.
- Key skills include detecting prodromes of illness by self-monitoring, and implementing an action plan appropriate to the developing risk.
- Adherence to prescribed medicines is an important objective of psychological treatment.
- Sequential interventions should be managed to achieve dose and durations adequate to allow definitive classification of outcomes as effective, ineffective or intolerable.
- Formal involvement of the family in psychoeducation for young patients appears to facilitate full recovery.
- Advising patients about decision-making and capacity to work is often an important part of the clinician's role.

**Key references**

American Psychiatric Association. Practice guideline for the treatment of patients with bipolar disorder (revision). *Am J Psychiatry* 2002;159(4 suppl):1–50.

Colom F, Vieta E, Martinez-Aran A et al. A randomized trial on the efficacy of group psychoeducation in the prophylaxis of recurrences in bipolar patients whose disease is in remission. *Arch Gen Psychiatry* 2003;60:402–7.

Cooper C, Bebbington P, King M et al. Why people do not take their psychotropic drugs as prescribed: results of the 2000 National Psychiatric Morbidity Survey. *Acta Psychiatr Scand* 2007;116:47–53.

Fisher R, Ury W, Patton B. *Getting to Yes: Negotiating Agreement Without Giving In*, 2nd edn. New York: Penguin, 1991.

Horne R, Weinman J. Patients' beliefs about prescribed medicines and their role in adherence to treatment in chronic physical illness. *J Psychosom Res* 1999;47:555–67.

Johnson RE, McFarland BH. Lithium use and discontinuation in a health maintenance organization. *Am J Psychiatry* 1996;153:993–1000.

Lam DH, Watkins ER, Hayward P et al. A randomized controlled study of cognitive therapy for relapse prevention for bipolar affective disorder – outcome of the first year. *Arch Gen Psychiatry* 2003;60: 145–52.

Leventhal H, Diefenbach M, Leventhal EA. Illness cognition: using common sense to understand treatment adherence and affect cognition interactions. *Cognit Ther Res* 1992;16:143–63.

Miklowitz DJ, George EL, Richards JA et al. A randomized study of family-focused psychoeducation and pharmacotherapy in the outpatient management of bipolar disorder. *Arch Gen Psychiatry* 2003;60: 904–12.

Nutt DJ, Sharpe M. Uncritical positive regard? Issues in the efficacy and safety of psychotherapy. *J Psychopharmacol* 2008;22:3–6.

Scott J, Paykel E, Morriss R et al. Cognitive-behavioural therapy for severe and recurrent bipolar disorders: randomised controlled trial. *Br J Psychiatry* 2006;188: 313–20.

Stone D, Patton B, Heen S, Fisher R. *Difficult Conversations. How to Discuss What Matters Most.* New York: Penguin, 2000.

Bipolar disorder often runs an episodic course and it is commonly thought of as a sequence of acute episodes of illness (mania, depression or mixed states) interspersed with euthymia. Short-term treatments are used in acute episodes, with the intention of discontinuing the medication on recovery. Long-term treatments are indefinite and are intended to prevent new episodes.

This simplified view of the illness is convenient and reflects clinical trial design. However, subsyndromal and a variety of chronic symptoms are common in bipolar disorder, and it is important to be aware of them. Indeed, in practice, they often drive treatment decisions. Chronic symptoms are usually related to anxiety, depression or cognition and are a disabling aspect of the long-term outcome. Unfortunately, there is little to guide the selection of treatment aimed at reducing the impact of these symptoms as they have almost never been the subject of clinical trials. What we can be most confident about is based on trials in bipolar I disorder and sometimes bipolar II disorder that address syndrome-level morbidity.

## Treatment options for mania and mixed states

Mania is often a medical emergency and carries appreciable risk for patients and those close to them. There are no reliable alternatives to treatment with medicines of proven efficacy. However, admission to hospital is itself associated with a subsequent fall in the level of symptoms. There are few specific measures that are recommended for the management of patients with mania and the most appropriate, ward milieu, has not been empirically established. Common sense suggests that a calming, uncrowded environment without overstimulation is likely to be best.

Figure 6.1 shows a flow chart derived from recommendations in the British Association for Psychopharmacology guidelines on the treatment of bipolar disorder. It outlines a simplified decision tree for mania and mixed episodes. The options are described in detail below.

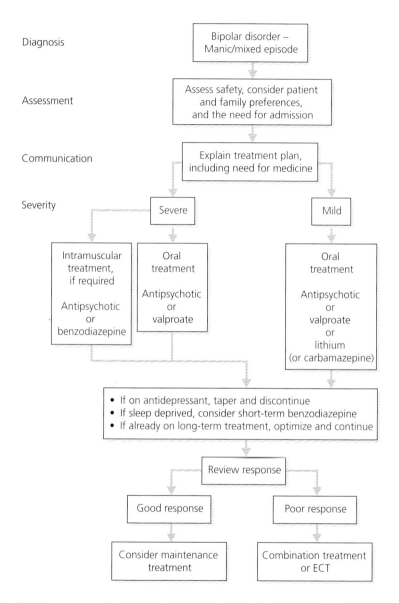

Diagnosis — Bipolar disorder – Manic/mixed episode

Assessment — Assess safety, consider patient and family preferences, and the need for admission

Communication — Explain treatment plan, including need for medicine

Severity — Severe | Mild

Intramuscular treatment, if required

Antipsychotic or benzodiazepine

Oral treatment

Antipsychotic or valproate

Oral treatment

Antipsychotic or valproate or lithium (or carbamazepine)

- If on antidepressant, taper and discontinue
- If sleep deprived, consider short-term benzodiazepine
- If already on long-term treatment, optimize and continue

Review response

Good response | Poor response

Consider maintenance treatment | Combination treatment or ECT

**Figure 6.1** Initial treatment scheme – mania and mixed states. ECT, electroconvulsive therapy. Adapted with permission from Goodwin GM. Evidence-based guidelines for treating bipolar disorder: recommendations from the British Association for Psychopharmacology. *J Psychopharmacol* 2003;17:149–73.

Drugs used in short-term treatment of acute mania and mixed states are summarized in Table 6.1.

**Antipsychotics.** Mania has long been treated with antipsychotic medicines. Indeed, at the start of the psychotropic era, chlorpromazine was first used with patients who had manic psychoses as well as those with schizophrenia. However, the efficacy of the older so-called typical antipsychotics was never examined in placebo-controlled trials. Instead, the short-term effect of acute tranquilization was probably taken to be self-evident. Indeed, the old term 'major tranquilizer' betrays the effect that was sought through sedation and even motor side effects – some clinicians used to refer approvingly to a 'chemical straitjacket'. Inevitably, such effects have often been associated with high doses and consequent severe adverse effects.

Pragmatic support for the use of an antipsychotic agent rather than lithium in severe mania came from a secondary analysis of data comparing generous doses of chlorpromazine and lithium. This suggested that the most activated manic patients were more effectively treated with chlorpromazine. The outcomes were realistic measures, such as the patient dropout rate and reduced nursing demands. Clinical practice has also tended to support the use of antipsychotics.

Antipsychotics are not merely sedative, they are also antimanic. This has been established by the results of recent trials examining the efficacy of the so-called atypical antipsychotics. The atypicals have a primary mode of action that is probably via blockade of dopamine receptors, although it remains controversial as to how the risk of extrapyramidal side effects (EPS) is reduced. It is a reasonable hypothesis that mania is a hyperdopaminergic state and that blockade of dopamine receptors represents an appropriate approach to treatment. Certainly, trials with aripiprazole, olanzapine, quetiapine, risperidone and ziprasidone now support the efficacy of atypical antipsychotics as a class in mania. Aripiprazole, olanzapine and ziprasidone are available in parenteral formulations for acute use and risperidone is available as a long-acting injectable formulation. Ziprasidone is not licensed in the UK.

Data from acute mania studies with the atypical antipsychotics are summarized in Figure 6.2. The reduction in the young mania rating

TABLE 6.1

**Drugs used in the short-term treatment of acute mania and mixed states**

| Class | Drug | Dose for uncompromised adult* (daily dose unless otherwise stated) |
|---|---|---|
| Typical antipsychotics (avoid EPS) | Chlorpromazine | • Oral: 300–1000 mg; tablets, syrup or suspension<br>• Intramuscular: 50 mg every 6–8 hours<br>• Per rectum: 100 mg every 6–8 hours |
| | Haloperidol | • Oral: 3–10 mg; tablets or liquid<br>• Intramuscular (or intravenous): 2–10 mg every 8 hours<br>• Depot (as decanoate): 50–100 mg per month |
| Atypical antipsychotics | Aripiprazole | • Oral: 15–30 mg; tablets<br>• Intramuscular: 5.25–15 mg (to a maximum of 30 mg per day) |
| | Asenapine | • Sublingual: 10–20 mg |
| | Clozapine | • Oral: 100–800 mg, taper in as tolerated; tablets |
| | Olanzapine | • Oral: 10–20 mg; tablets or oro-dispersible<br>• Intramuscular: 5–10 mg (20 mg maximum) as up to 3 injections per 24 hours |
| | Quetiapine | • Oral: 200–800 mg, taper in (average dose 600 mg); tablets |
| | Risperidone | • Oral: 3–6 mg; tablets or liquid<br>• Depot: 25–50 mg every 2 weeks |
| | Ziprasidone | • Oral: 80–160 mg; tablets<br>• Intramuscular: 10–20 mg every 4 hours (to a maximum of 40 mg) |

CONTINUED

TABLE 6.1 (CONTINUED)

| | | |
|---|---|---|
| Anti-convulsants | Valproate | • Oral: 750–2500 mg as semisodium, tablets; increase by 30% for sodium valproate |
| | Carbamazepine | • Oral: taper up to 1200 mg; tablets |
| | Oxcarbazepine | • Oral: taper up to 1200 mg; tablets |
| Lithium | Lithium carbonate (note formulations have different bioavailability) | • Oral: 400–1800 mg as tablets; 500–300 mg as liquid according to blood level (> 1 and < 1.5 mmol/L for mania) |
| | Lithium citrate | • Oral: 500–3000 mg according to blood level; liquid |
| Benzo-diazepines | Lorazepam | • Oral: 4–16 mg in divided doses; tablets<br>• Intravenous slowly into a large vein: 2–4 mg every 6–8 hours |
| | Clonazepam | • Oral: 2–8 mg in divided doses; tablets<br>• Intravenous slowly into a large vein: 1 mg every 6–8 hours |

*Reduce dose in the elderly or if otherwise indicated.
EPS, extrapyramidal side effects.

scale is presented as a global effect, but in all these trials changes occurred on almost every item of the scale, not just on those related to sedation. Haloperidol has also been included as a comparator in a number of placebo-controlled studies and in some head-to-head comparators. The results confirm that haloperidol at doses of around 10 mg has antimanic actions comparable to the atypical medications.

Asenapine is a new addition to the atypical antipsychotics. It has an antimanic action like the other medications, but has a different sublingual route of administration, which in some circumstances may be preferred (e.g. for patients who will not swallow tablets).

EPS are manifest as akathisia, parkinsonism or dystonia during acute treatment, and patients with bipolar disorder are probably more likely

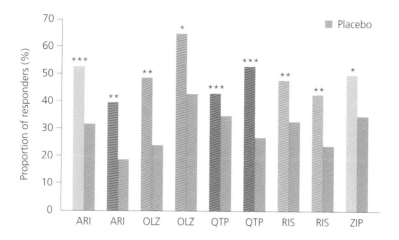

**Figure 6.2** Summary of data from acute studies of mania with atypical antipsychotics. The treatment effects are shown as the percentages of patients achieving 50% or greater decrease from the baseline score on the young mania rating scale (YMRS) at 3 weeks for aripiprazole (ARI), olanzapine (OLZ), quetiapine (QTP), risperidone (RIS) and ziprasidone (ZIP) compared with placebo. In each trial, the active treatment was shown to be significantly superior to placebo; *$p < 0.05$; **$p \leq 0.01$; ***$p \leq 0.001$ compared with placebo. Data are from Sachs et al. *J Psychopharmacol* 2006;20:536–46. Keck et al. *Am J Psychiatry* 2003;160:1651–8; Tohen et al. *Am J Psychiatry* 1999;156:702–9; Tohen et al. *Arch Gen Psychiatry* 2000;57:841–9; Bowden et al. *J Clin Psych* 2005;66:111–21; McIntyre et al. *Eur Neuropsychopharmacol* 2005;15:573–85; Smulevich et al. *Eur Neuropsychopharmacol* 2005;15:75–84; Hirschfeld et al. *Am J Psychiatry* 2004;161:1057–65; Keck et al. *Am J Psychiatry* 2003;160:741–8.

to show acute EPS when treated with comparable doses of haloperidol than those with schizophrenia. There are two important clinical disadvantages to this. First, the subjective experience of EPS, especially akathisia and dystonia, may be highly aversive and produce a negative attitude in patients towards subsequent treatment of their illness with any sort of medicine. Secondly, naturalistic studies in schizophrenia suggest that development of acute EPS is predictive of subsequent tardive dyskinesia. The most important clinical message is that antimanic action can be achieved without EPS and the improved therapeutic ratio of the atypical antipsychotics makes this more likely.

With the success in reducing EPS has come an increased emphasis on weight gain and metabolic disturbance attributable to antipsychotic medicines when addressing the risk/benefit for different agents. Weight gain is a particular problem of long-term treatment, but also occurs early in treatment, and it should not be ignored.

There is international support for the use of antipsychotics as first-line agents for mania and this is reflected by the advice contained in a number of recent guidelines.

**Valproate, lithium and carbamazepine.** The seminal randomized, placebo-controlled trial of valproate in acute mania in the 1990s was the catalyst for major changes in the treatment of bipolar disorder. This trial not only showed that valproate is an effective antimanic agent, but also that lithium appears to have comparable efficacy. Valproate is a generic term used to describe the several formulations of valproic acid, which is the presumed active chemical entity. Sodium valproate is widely used in epilepsy and is available as a sustained-release preparation. Valproate semisodium (divalproex in North America) is a non-covalent dimer molecule that has been produced in several formulations (best known as Depakote), including a slow-release form. In bipolar disorder, valproate has been studied almost exclusively as valproate semisodium. Valproate is effective in severe (including psychotic) mania. Aggressive dosing to achieve serum levels effective against mania (> 80 µg/mL) may result in acute gastrointestinal side effects, tremor, sedation or cognitive impairment, but does not produce EPS.

Lithium was initially discovered to be an antimanic agent by Cade in 1947, based on changes observed in chronically manic patients and early crossover trials. Satisfactory confirmatory data from trials employing modern methodology, such as parallel-group design, formal rating scales and statistical analysis, were not available until 1995. Lithium monotherapy is generally preferred for the treatment of less severe manic states.

There is also limited evidence to support the efficacy of carbamazepine in mania, but it is seldom advocated as first-line treatment. Oxcarbazepine is a distinct but related chemical entity with much the same pharmacokinetic interactions as carbamazepine (see 'Combination treatment' below). Its efficacy in mania is imputed from the evidence for carbamazepine, but controlled trial data establishing efficacy have not been published. In one study, oxcarbazepine was no better than placebo for reducing manic symptoms in children and adolescents with bipolar I disorder.

**Other drugs.** Gabapentin, lamotrigine, oxcarbazepine and topiramate (all anticonvulsants) are ineffective in acute mania. Unproven and ineffective treatments are not acceptable alternatives to agents shown to be effective for acute mania in randomized controlled trials.

**Combination treatment.** Episodes of mania occur commonly in patients who are already taking lithium or valproate as a long-term treatment. In such cases, it is common to add an antipsychotic to lithium or valproate. This strategy is supported by trials in which atypical antipsychotics or haloperidol in combination with lithium or valproate proved superior to monotherapy with either lithium or valproate.

These findings underpin the current advice of the American Psychiatric Association, which also recommends combining lithium or valproate with an antipsychotic in patients who are not already receiving long-term treatment. It clearly makes sense when there is reason to spare the antipsychotic dose and/or long-term treatment with lithium or valproate is planned. However, adherence is such a major issue that the initiation of long-term treatment when patients are manic may not be a good strategy unless the attitude of the patient when well is already known.

Carbamazepine is not an ideal agent for combination treatment because it induces the synthesis of liver enzymes and this reduces its levels and those of many other drugs. Oxcarbazepine induces the same enzyme systems as carbamazepine and reduces levels of the same drugs. However, as oxcarbazepine itself is metabolized by a different pathway, its own level is not affected.

**Benzodiazepines** are not believed to be antimanic. They are used adjunctively with other agents and may be required when sedation or tranquilization is a priority (e.g. after a prolonged period of sleep deprivation). Benzodiazepines are safe and have few important pharmacokinetic interactions with other agents. Their use may also reduce the required doses of antipsychotics or other drugs.

## Strategy for treating mania

The objective in treating mania is to control behavioral disturbance and shorten the duration of the episode. Where possible, the treatment should be agreed with the patient, and thought should be given to creating advance directives that may facilitate future treatment. Antipsychotics or valproate, as monotherapy or in combination, are the preferred options. However, avoidance of EPS is also a priority. This argues for minimal doses of classic antipsychotics if used, a low threshold for the preferential use of valproate or atypical antipsychotics, careful monitoring of clinical response and appropriate laboratory monitoring. Restoration of the sleep–wake cycle, if greatly disturbed, is an early objective.

Benzodiazepines should be withdrawn once their desired effect on sleep has been obtained. Antipsychotic agents should be continued until full remission of acute symptoms has been achieved (up to 2–3 months). There should be an early emphasis on understanding the patient's attitude to treatment in the long term, and clinicians must be aware of the risk of a switch to depression. It is not well established which treatments make such a switch more likely; two small studies suggest that the risk may be higher with typical than atypical antipsychotics.

## Short-term treatments and mixed states

Mixed states may be slower to resolve during acute treatment than more classic mania. There have been no studies to determine the optimal treatment for this subgroup by comparison with other manic presentations. In view of the actions of some atypical antipsychotics on mania and depression (see below), it might be anticipated that quetiapine or olanzapine, for example, might be the most logical choices; however, there are no data showing that any specific antipsychotic has an advantage compared with another in mixed states. There is no reason to start or continue treatment with an antidepressant in a mixed state when the predominant affect is mania.

**Electroconvulsive therapy (ECT) in refractory mania and mixed states.** Audit studies suggest that ECT is a highly effective treatment for mania, with response rates of over 80%. Given its established effects on severe depression, ECT might also be expected to work well in mixed states, although there are no randomized controlled trials to support the use of ECT in mania or mixed states. It is clearly an option for those patients who express a preference for it, when mania is refractory to drug treatment and in women with severe mania during pregnancy, when drug treatment may be undesirable. It is, of course, more usual for ECT to be considered for the treatment of depression in bipolar patients.

## Treatment options for depressive episodes

Patients with bipolar disorder will, on average, spend more of their time depressed than in manic or mixed states. It is therefore surprising that the treatment of bipolar depression has been relatively neglected until quite recently and there is a paucity of evidence from randomized trials to demonstrate the efficacy or relative effectiveness of different approaches to relieving depressive symptoms. Nevertheless, opinion changes and the negative sentiment against antidepressants in bipolar depression has hardened in the wake of adverse media coverage of antidepressant use in general, the limited evidence of efficacy in bipolar depression and the perceived association with switch or mood instability when used as monotherapy. Quetiapine and lamotrigine are now more likely to be used as first-line agents for many patients. This change will shift the risk–benefit analysis as quetiapine is associated with adverse metabolic effects and lamotrigine has a low but real risk of severe rash and even potentially fatal Stevens–Johnson syndrome.

Figure 6.3 shows a flow chart derived from recommendations in the British Association for Psychopharmacology guideline for the treatment of bipolar depressive episodes. Table 6.2 lists drugs used in the short-term treatment of acute depressive states. The options are described in more detail below.

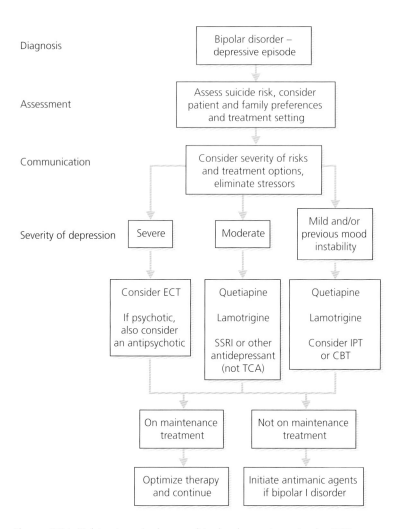

**Figure 6.3** Initial treatment scheme – bipolar depressive episode. CBT, cognitive–behavior therapy; ECT, electroconvulsive therapy; IPT, interpersonal therapy; SSRI, selective serotonin reuptake inhibitor; TCA, tricyclic antidepressant. Adapted with permission from Goodwin GM. Evidence-based guidelines for treating bipolar disorder: recommendations from the British Association for Psychopharmacology. *J Psychopharmacol* 2003;17:149–73.

**Antidepressants.** Compared with the evidence for the effectiveness of antidepressants in unipolar disorder, the available data relating

TABLE 6.2

**Drugs used in the short-term treatment of acute depressive states**

| Class | Drug | Daily dose for uncompromised adult* |
|---|---|---|
| Antidepressants: SSRIs | Citalopram | 20–60 mg; tablets or oral drops |
| | Escitalopram (isomer) | 10–20 mg; tablets |
| | Sertraline | 100–200 mg; tablets |
| | Fluoxetine | 10–40 mg; tablets or liquid |
| | Paroxetine | 20–60 mg; tablets or liquid |
| | Fluvoxamine | 100–300 mg; tablets |
| Antidepressants: other | Bupropion | 150–450 mg; tablets |
| Antidepressants: MAOIs | Moclobemide | 300–600 mg; tablets |
| | Tranylcypromine | 10–40 mg; tablets |
| | Phenelzine | 30–75 mg; tablets |
| Anticonvulsants | Lamotrigine | 100–400 mg; tablets, taper in slowly (see SPC) |
| | Valproate | See Table 6.1: little to guide dosing |
| Atypical antipsychotics | Quetiapine | 300–600 mg; tablets, start at lower doses |
| | Olanzapine | 5–20 mg used in varying combinations with fluoxetine, 25–75 mg, in USA |
| Lithium | See Table 6.1 | Choose level > 0.5 mmol/L, according to tolerability |

*Reduce dose in the elderly or if otherwise indicated.
MAOIs, monoamine oxidase inhibitors; SPC, summary of product characteristics; SSRIs, selective serotonin reuptake inhibitors.

specifically to bipolar depression are extremely limited. The Systematic Treatment Enhancement Program for Bipolar Disorder (STEP-BD) study found no advantage for the adjunctive use of paroxetine or bupropion compared with placebo. In another three-arm study in bipolar depression, paroxetine monotherapy was not significantly more effective than placebo, but quetiapine was superior to placebo. The only high-quality study supporting the efficacy of any single standard antidepressant agent found fluoxetine and olanzapine to be superior to olanzapine alone. It is not known whether this represents a benefit that generalizes to combining fluoxetine with other antipsychotics or whether olanzapine would augment the effect of other standard antidepressants. The availability of data from recent well-powered double-blind trials lessens the need to extrapolate from meta-analysis of small studies, which supports an overall benefit for standard antidepressant medications as a class.

There are no grounds at present for recommending one antidepressant over another on the basis of efficacy, although fluoxetine and monoamine oxidase inhibitors are probably the best supported by the existing evidence (which is derived from small or poor-quality studies).

Antidepressants, if used, are best combined with an agent that will reduce the risk of mania (such as lithium, valproate or an antipsychotic).

**ECT** is effective in severe depression and the randomized trials of ECT have included patients with bipolar disorder, although no studies have concentrated exclusively on ECT in these groups. Systematic review of ECT data supports its general efficacy and also its relatively greater efficacy compared with antidepressants. The adverse consequence of memory disturbance may not be dissociable from effective dosing, but it is usually mild. The use of ECT is tempered by the continuing unfavorable portrayal of the treatment by the media, and anecdotal reports of severe, but largely unexplained, subjective side effects such as loss of identity, complete amnesia and inability to read. The most extravagant claims about the adverse effects of ECT appear less likely to be due to the treatment than to other grievances in the minds of the claimants. Access to ECT will continue to be necessary because it offers such an effective way of relieving severe and dangerous depressive states.

**Lithium.** Evidence for the acute efficacy of lithium in bipolar depression is generally inadequate; early trials were all small crossover studies of short duration. The largest double-blind study including lithium monotherapy for bipolar depression found no benefit of lithium over placebo. It is also emerging from systematic review of the trials of long-term treatment that the efficacy of lithium in preventing depressive relapse is modest, and less than its efficacy against mania. Nevertheless, lithium occupies a prominent place in many treatment guidelines, which express expert preference for the use of lithium rather than antidepressants as first-line treatment for bipolar depression. The conflict between opinion and evidence highlights an area of considerable uncertainty. It would be helpful if lithium is included as a key comparator in new monotherapy studies of compounds developed for use specifically in bipolar disorder.

**Anticonvulsants.** Because of their reputation as 'mood stabilizers', the anticonvulsants carbamazepine and valproate are often advocated for use in acute depression, although the evidence supporting their antidepressant efficacy is almost non-existent.

Lamotrigine, which has an entirely different mechanism of action, is the only anticonvulsant compound for which there is good evidence supporting a significant clinical benefit in acute bipolar depression. It does not increase the risk of switching to a manic state.

**Antipsychotics** have long had a place in the management of psychotic depression but their more routine use in the treatment of bipolar depression is an emerging development. Olanzapine appears to be a modest antidepressant in bipolar depression but it has a greater effect when combined with fluoxetine. The serotonergic actions of some of the atypical antipsychotics may make them unusually efficacious in depressed states. Indeed, the data for quetiapine in bipolar depression have been particularly interesting because of the large scale of the trials, the strong apparent benefit and the consistency of effect in a variety of subgroups (bipolar I and II, rapid cycling, severe depression). The unusual status of quetiapine was recognized in October 2006, when it became the only drug approved by the US Food and Drug Administration as monotherapy for bipolar depression; the combination of olanzapine and fluoxetine has also been approved.

The properties of quetiapine that underpin these effects are not fully understood but they do not appear to be the result of a class effect shared by atypical antipsychotics. Differential antidepressant efficacy of agents in this class is suggested by controlled studies involving aripiprazole, bifeprunox and risperidone, which have not produced encouraging results.

## Treatment-emergent mania following depression

Just like the switch from mania to depression, a switch from depression to mania may be a consequence of either the course of the illness or the treatment; some treatments may have a greater propensity to cause switching than others. Both in practice and in theory, it is difficult to disentangle whether or not mania has been triggered by drug treatment. The long-standing controversy around the potential of standard antidepressants to induce mania is constrained by considerably better data than were available just a few years ago. Only randomized placebo-controlled trials that include measures of mood elevation can establish whether certain drugs increase the probability of switching. Meta-analysis has shown that a manic event is two to three times more likely to occur during treatment with tricyclic antidepressants than during treatment with selective serotonin reuptake inhibitors or placebo. Coadministration of an antimanic agent can, however, reduce this risk. In a study lacking placebo control, Post and colleagues found significantly higher rates of treatment-emergent hypomania or mania in depressed bipolar participants receiving adjunctive venlafaxine than in those randomized to other antidepressant comparators (bupropion and sertraline). Combined noradrenergic and serotonergic action may be particularly likely to induce a switch.

## Strategy for treating depression: when short term becomes long term

The imperative of offering proven treatments brings lamotrigine, quetiapine and olanzapine to mind as first-line options. As depression is so often a long-term problem, effective short-term treatment often becomes long term. Therefore, it makes sense preferentially to offer interventions with both short- and long-term efficacy. Almost by default, quetiapine and lamotrigine become first-line interventions owing to the data supporting their efficacy in preventing relapse in the long term, as described below.

In contrast, it is usually recommended that antidepressants be discontinued after the acute resolution of symptoms. The belief that all antidepressants generally destabilize the course of the illness in bipolar patients is not consistent with available data. In fact, the little controlled data that are available indicate that destabilization is just as likely to result from discontinuation of antidepressants after recovery. The only evidence that antidepressants worsen outcomes is in rapid-cycling patients.

When antidepressants are discontinued, it is recommended that the dose is tapered off over 4 weeks, if possible. Antidepressants may be discontinued more quickly if patients develop mania.

Refractory depression is not uncommon. Unfortunately, there are not data from randomized trials to guide practice. In the absence of specific guidelines for the management of refractory bipolar depression, treatment can follow recommendations for refractory depression in general.

Whether the treatment of depression in patients with bipolar spectrum disorder should be different from that in patients with unipolar disorder remains uncertain. Depressed bipolar patients with concurrent sub-syndromal manic symptoms do appear to be at high risk of worsening symptoms when treated with standard antidepressant medications.

**Key points – short-term treatments**

- The objective of short-term treatment is to reduce the severity and shorten the duration of an acute episode.
- Antipsychotics, valproate, carbamazepine and lithium are antimanic. The clinical context and, whenever possible, patient preference and experience should determine the choice.
- Antipsychotics may be preferred in highly active or agitated patients with mania. Extrapyramidal side effects (EPS) should be avoided if possible. Valproate is also effective in severe mania.

**Key points – short-term treatments** *continued*

- The atypical antipsychotics (aripiprazole, asenapine, olanzapine, quetiapine, risperidone and ziprasidone) have shown efficacy as monotherapy in placebo-controlled trials in mania and are less likely to produce EPS than, for example, haloperidol.
- Combining an antipsychotic with lithium or valproate can facilitate the acute treatment response. Combinations with aripiprazole, asenapine, haloperidol, olanzapine, quetiapine or risperidone have been shown to be superior to lithium or valproate alone, especially when mania recurs on maintenance therapy.
- Benzodiazepines can induce sedation and regularize sleep when added to antimanic agents. They should be discontinued after the desired response is established.
- Short-term treatments for mania can be discontinued after full remission of symptoms (usually 2–3 months).
- A switch from mania to depression may occur in the course of the illness. There is limited evidence that the atypical antipsychotics may be less likely to provoke this than the older typical antipsychotics.
- Electroconvulsive therapy provides an important treatment option for manic or mixed states resistant to treatment or arising in pregnancy, and for severe depression.
- Quetiapine and lamotrigine are important options for treating bipolar depression.
- Antidepressants may be effective for treating some cases of depression in bipolar disorder, but are best used in combination with an agent that will reduce the risk of mania (lithium, valproate or an antipsychotic).
- The risk of a switch from depression to mania is greater with dual-action drugs such as tricyclic antidepressants or venlafaxine than with other antidepressants (particularly SSRIs).
- The available data support avoidance or discontinuation of antidepressant medication for rapid-cycling patients.

# Key references

Bhagwagar Z, Goodwin GM. The role of lithium in the treatment of bipolar depression. *Clin Neurosci Res* 2002;2:222–7.

Bottlender R, Rudolf D, Strauss A, Möller HJ. Mood-stabilizers reduce the risk of developing antidepressant-induced maniform states in acute treatment of bipolar I depressed patients. *J Affect Disord* 2001; 63:79–83.

Bowden CL, Brugger AM, Swann AC et al. Efficacy of divalproex vs lithium and placebo in the treatment of mania. *JAMA* 1994;271:918–24.

Gijsman HJ, Geddes JR, Rendell JM et al. Antidepressants for bipolar depression: a systematic review of randomized, controlled trials. *Am J Psychiatry* 2004;161:1537–47.

Goodwin GM. Evidence-based guidelines for treating bipolar disorder: recommendations from the British Association for Psychopharmacology. *J Psychopharmacol* 2003;17:149–73.

Mukherjee S, Sackeim HA, Schnur DB. Electroconvulsive therapy of acute manic episodes: a review of 50 years' experience. *Am J Psychiatry* 1994;151:169–76.

Müller-Oerlinghausen B, Retzow A, Henn FA et al. Valproate as an adjunct to neuroleptic medication for the treatment of acute episodes of mania: a prospective, randomized, double-blind, placebo-controlled, multicenter study. *J Clin Psychopharmacol* 2000;20:195–203.

Peet M. Induction of mania with selective serotonin re-uptake inhibitors and tricyclic antidepressants. *Br J Psychiatry* 1994;164:549–50.

Post RM, Altshuler LL, Leverich GS et al. Mood switch in bipolar depression: comparison of adjunctive venlafaxine, bupropion and sertraline. *Br J Psychiatry* 2006; 189:124–31.

Prien RF, Caffey E-M Jr, Klett CJ. Comparison of lithium carbonate and chlorpromazine in the treatment of mania. Report of the Veterans Administration and National Institute of Mental Health Collaborative Study Group. *Arch Gen Psychiatry* 1972;26:146–53.

Sachs GS, Nierenberg AA, Calabrese JR et al. Effectiveness of adjunctive antidepressant treatment for bipolar depression. *N Engl J Med* 2007;356: 1711–22.

Sachs GS, Printz DJ, Kahn DA et al. The Expert Consensus Guideline Series: Medication Treatment of Bipolar Disorder 2000. *Postgrad Med* 2000;spec no:1–104.

Schneck CD, Miklowitz DJ, Miyahara S et al. The prospective course of rapid-cycling bipolar disorder: findings from the STEP-BD. *Am J Psychiatry* 2008;165: 370–7.

Smith LA, Cornelius V, Warnock A et al. Acute bipolar mania: a systematic review and meta-analysis of co-therapy vs. monotherapy. *Acta Psychiatr Scand* 2007;115:12–20.

Smith LA, Cornelius V, Warnock A et al. Pharmacological interventions for acute bipolar mania: a systematic review of randomized placebo-controlled trials. *Bipolar Disord* 2007;9:551–60.

The UK ECT Review Group. Efficacy and safety of electroconvulsive therapy in depressive disorders: a systematic review and meta-analysis. *Lancet* 2003;361:799–808.

Wagner KD, Kowatch RA, Emslie GJ et al. A double-blind, randomized, placebo-controlled trial of oxcarbazepine in the treatment of bipolar disorder in children and adolescents. *Am J Psychiatry* 2006;163:1179–86.

Weisler RH, Calabrese JR, Thase ME et al. Efficacy of quetiapine monotherapy for the treatment of depressive episodes in bipolar I disorder: a post hoc analysis of combined results from 2 double-blind, randomized, placebo-controlled studies. *J Clin Psychiatry* 2008;69:769–82.

The objective of long-term treatment in bipolar disorder is to reduce the risk of relapse, suicide and overall mortality. This can also be referred to as mood stabilization; drugs with efficacy against both manic and depressive relapse are often described as mood stabilizers.

The term mood stabilizer is a functional one that conveniently describes a group of otherwise pharmacologically different agents, rather like the term antipsychotic or antidepressant. Unfortunately, it has been bestowed indiscriminately on some anticonvulsants such as gabapentin and topiramate, with little evidence to support efficacy against relapse. By contrast, the atypical antipsychotic quetiapine has been shown to prevent relapse to mania or depression and therefore is a mood stabilizer. In fact, the long-term use of a variety of agents alone or in combination may contribute to mood stability. More neutral terminology often seems prudent.

In unipolar disorder, relapse (the return of symptoms treated in an acute episode) is often distinguished from recurrence (the re-appearance of symptoms after the sustained remission of an index episode). This distinction is not useful in bipolar disorder, where episodes are often frequent. We will therefore refer to long-term treatment for prevention of relapse.

Figure 7.1 shows the long-term treatment scheme based on the British Association for Psychopharmacology guidelines. The main medications used in the long-term management of bipolar disorder are listed in Table 7.1 (see page 96), together with some of the issues relating to safety.

## Long-term treatment with lithium

Lithium is the classic long-term treatment for bipolar I disorder. Adequate, but not large, numbers of patients have been studied in placebo-controlled trials. Over 1 year, relapse rates in patients receiving lithium were 40% compared with 61% in those receiving placebo; the relative risk reduction remained constant at 33% over 2–3 years.

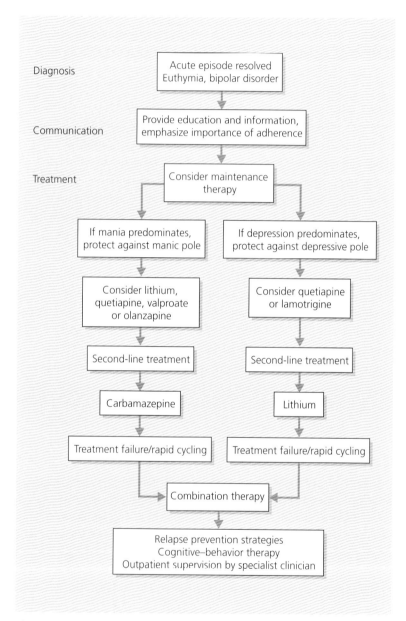

**Figure 7.1** Long-term treatment scheme – maintenance therapy. Adapted with permission from Goodwin GM. Evidence-based guidelines for treating bipolar disorder: recommendations from the British Association for Psychopharmacology. *J Psychopharmacol* 2003;17:149–73.

Patients who do well on lithium for this time period appear to continue to do well with continued treatment in the longer term.

In the prevention of relapse, lithium is probably more effective against mania than against depression (relative risk reduction of 40% vs 23%, respectively). Plasma lithium levels below 0.5 mmol/L are usually too low to be effective and levels over 0.8 mmol/L are often recommended. However, achieving high levels in the face of significant side effects is likely to be counterproductive. The highest dose that produces minimal side effects should therefore be used.

## Long-term treatment with antipsychotics

Classic antipsychotics have often been used as a long-term treatment in bipolar patients, sometimes in depot formulations. Their place is poorly established, however, because of very limited evidence from clinical trials and concerns about tardive dyskinesia.

The atypical antipsychotics have been the subject of intense recent study. Companies seeking to extend their product licenses for the treatment of schizophrenia to bipolar disorder have provided a mass of new data. Following response in acute mania, aripiprazole and olanzapine have been shown to be effective in the long term in placebo-controlled studies of relapse prevention. Like lithium, both appear to be more effective in preventing manic relapse than depressive relapse. Quetiapine, in confirmation of its unusual acute efficacy in bipolar depression, has been shown to prevent relapse to mania or depression, irrespective of the pole of the acute index episode, both as monotherapy and in combination with lithium or valproate.

Antipsychotic agents may often be appropriate for the long-term management of bipolar patients in whom psychotic features are prominent. In addition, clozapine, used in combination with 'usual treatment' with lithium or anticonvulsants, has been shown to be superior to 'usual treatment' alone over 1 year in patients with treatment-resistant bipolar disorder, including those with rapid cycling and mixed states.

## Long-term treatment with anticonvulsants

Anticonvulsants are often described quite uncritically as mood stabilizers. In part, this reflects the hypothesis that they work against an underlying 'instability' that has something in common with epilepsy. While this concept is heuristically useful, it is unlikely to be true. Anticonvulsants prevent seizures, but there is no evidence that they reverse the primary neuronal instability in epilepsy. Unlike the case with the antipsychotics for mania, the evidence does not support a class effect for anticonvulsants in any phase of bipolar disorder. There are adequate long-term data to support the use of individual anticonvulsants.

**Valproate** (as valproate semisodium) has been studied in a single long-term, randomized controlled trial, which was underpowered for its primary endpoint. Rates of relapse were 24% for valproate and 38% for placebo. While the difference is not statistically significant, it suggests a relative risk reduction of 37%, which is numerically comparable to that with lithium. It is not possible to say whether valproate has a greater efficacy against manic than against depressive relapse.

Despite this statistically weak evidence base, valproate is used widely in North America and increasingly in other countries. It has a reputation for better tolerability than lithium – certainly when lithium is used at doses that produce plasma levels over 0.8 mmol/L. However, it is not without adverse effects, particularly weight gain. Valproate is also associated with an increased risk of polycystic ovarian syndrome.

**Carbamazepine** was the first anticonvulsant to be advocated for the long-term treatment of bipolar disorder. However, it has been shown to be inferior to lithium in preventing relapse.

**Lamotrigine** has a novel profile in relapse prevention. It is more effective against depression than mania. Two long-term trials have compared lithium and lamotrigine with placebo, one in patients with a recent depressive episode and the other in patients with a recent manic episode. The findings were essentially the same in both studies. Overall, the benefit was similar for lithium and lamotrigine but the largest effect of lithium was on manic relapse and the greatest effect of lamotrigine was on depression.

## Long-term treatment with antidepressants

Antidepressant monotherapy is not recommended in patients with bipolar I disorder. A small but highly regarded study conducted more than 20 years ago cast a negative perspective on long-term antidepressant treatment. First, it showed that imipramine alone resulted in an unacceptable number of manic relapses over a 1–2-year follow-up period; this effect was prevented by co-treatment with lithium. Second, the combination of imipramine with lithium was only a little more effective than lithium alone in preventing depressive relapse. It remains uncertain whether or not antidepressants should be used long term in bipolar disorder, even in conjunction with other agents, because there have been no systematic large-scale studies to clarify the issue since this initial study. Given the significant burden of disease imposed by chronic depressive symptoms and recurrent depressive episodes, this may appear surprising.

The long-term treatment of bipolar I disorder with antidepressants is, however, common in clinical practice. Data from STEP-BD and the Stanley Bipolar Network suggest that relatively few patients enjoy long-term benefit with antidepressants. Audit evidence, however, generally supports continuing successful long-term prophylaxis with antidepressants in bipolar patients who are also receiving lithium, valproate, carbamazepine or antipsychotics.

Patients with bipolar II disorder and, in particular, those with bipolar spectrum depression, have not been sufficiently investigated. It is possible that effective treatment with antidepressants can be achieved without adding an antimanic agent. This area merits further investigation as the diagnostic issues become more clearly defined.

## Long-term combination therapy

The early discovery of lithium and its initial status as something of a 'wonder drug' perhaps exaggerated our perceptions of the effectiveness of lithium monotherapy. In fact, no more than 30% of patients started on lithium do well over a 5-year follow-up period. A principle in other areas of medicine is that the combination of two partially effective treatments may make a potent treatment. The same approach is now developing in bipolar disorder. In our view, it would be preferable to base practice on systematic audit and, preferably, randomized trials of particular combinations. Combination treatment can too quickly become bizarre polypharmacy and even pose a danger to patients.

Systematic study of combinations of currently available medicines appears increasingly necessary because of the intensifying pressure to intervene early in the natural history of bipolar disorder. Effective prevention of disease progression may require combination therapy from as early in the illness course as possible. We are uncertain what combination, if any, to recommend after a first episode. To resolve the key uncertainties, there is widespread support for large simple trials in bipolar disorder. Such trials require the creation of adequate capacity in the form of collaborative networks of clinicians who can incorporate simple trial methods into everyday clinical practice.

## Suicide

Suicide is a major long-term risk for patients with bipolar I disorder and contributes disproportionately to their increased mortality. Long-term follow-up of patients identified by admission to hospital (the most severely affected group) show suicide rates to be around 10%. Suicide is associated with depression and mixed states. Therefore, successful long-term treatment has the potential to reduce the risk of suicide by preventing new episodes or reducing chronic symptoms. Naturalistic studies suggest that suicide rates are lower in patients who receive long-term treatment. In STEP-BD, for 3721 patients with 5642 patient-years of follow-up, the rate of suicide attempts was 4.6 per 1000 patient-years and the completed suicide rate was 1.4 per 1000 patient-years.

Whether lithium has particular efficacy as an anti-suicide agent is an important question that has not been addressed in a full-scale randomized trial. A recently reported case–control study from STEP-BD did not find evidence of a protective effect of lithium, but meta-analysis of randomized studies and naturalistic datasets did.

## Stopping long-term treatment

Discontinuation of long-term treatment is not indicated when there is good clinical control of the illness. When necessary, doses should be tapered off, particularly in the case of lithium where there is a specific risk of manic relapse. Poor compliance is a contraindication to prescribing lithium because of the risk of new illness episodes on discontinuation.

## Adverse effects of long-term treatment

Adverse effects certainly contribute to poor adherence to prescribed treatment and may pose dangers in their own right. The increase in treatment options for the long term and the common use of combinations pose new challenges for the field. In addition, this arises on a background of increased obesity within the population of most developed countries and a growing realization that bipolar patients may be at high risk for a variety of physical health problems.

**Weight gain** has long been the most important problem associated with many of the long-term drug treatments such as lithium, valproate and the tricyclic antidepressants. Weight gain is not just a cosmetic issue; it is associated with a constellation of changes sometimes described as the metabolic syndrome. This includes abdominal obesity, adverse blood lipid profiles, glucose intolerance and hypertension, all of which are risk factors for cardiovascular disease and stroke. Glucose intolerance is the forerunner to type 2 diabetes. Risk of complications at a given level of obesity depends importantly on racial background. Patients of Indian background, for example, are at risk above a body mass index (BMI) of 25, in contrast with Caucasians for whom the equivalent point is 30.

The atypical antipsychotics, particularly clozapine, olanzapine and quetiapine, (although no antipsychotic is entirely excluded except ziprasidone) appear independently to contribute to these risks. Their use increases the need for monitoring of physical health indices and treating where appropriate. In addition, there is concern that the antipsychotics may increase the risk of acute ketoacidosis by other, as yet poorly understood, mechanisms. Greater vigilance for the physical welfare of bipolar patients is necessary. Numerous recommendations for monitoring schedules have been advocated and are worthy of consideration, although none is evidence based. Waist circumference, weight (BMI), vital signs and serum lipids are likely to be the most

89

sensitive indicators of treatment-emergent metabolic risk, and these should be monitored routinely. Switching between antipsychotics to reduce the burden of metabolic side effects should also be considered.

**Tardive dyskinesia** has long been, and remains, a concern for patients treated with antipsychotics in the long term. Development of acute EPS appears to predict an increased risk of tardive dyskinesia, and bipolar patients may be at a slightly greater risk of motor side effects when taking antipsychotics than are patients with schizophrenia.

Avoidance of EPS is an indication to use atypical antipsychotics because they have a more favorable therapeutic ratio than classic antipsychotics. There are also differences between the atypical antipsychotics: for example, quetiapine and clozapine have an intrinsically lower capacity to occupy dopamine receptors than olanzapine and risperidone; increasing the dose of olanzapine and risperidone will produce motor effects, while increasing the dose of quetiapine and clozapine will not.

**Hyperprolactinemia.** There is a related concern about prolactin elevation with some antipsychotics, especially those with high affinity for dopamine $D_2$ receptors. This has long been associated with the typical antipsychotics but is also seen with risperidone, for example. Hyperprolactinemia produces a hypogonadal state which is most marked in women. In the long term, this can predispose to bone demineralization and fractures. Antipsychotics with a lower affinity for $D_2$ receptors, such as clozapine and quetiapine, and the partial agonist aripiprazole are less likely to cause such problems in long-term treatment.

The increasing use of atypical antipsychotics in long-term treatment will complicate the medical management of bipolar patients. These problems and the additional burden of adverse effects that comes with combination treatments will require a careful balancing of risk and benefits. Monitoring is already established because of lithium use, but how the long-term problems of lithium use should be weighed against those of, for example, quetiapine remains uncertain.

## Prescribing in pregnancy and after childbirth

One of the more common clinical dilemmas arises when a woman with bipolar disorder wishes to become, or is already, pregnant. The decision of whether or not to stop long-term treatment is reached by balancing clinical priorities, and will depend on the patient's preferences and past history. There is therefore no simple rule.

The potential benefits of compliance with long-term treatment during pregnancy are that the patient remains symptom-free and enjoys normal bonding with the child. The risk of major congenital malformations in the general population is 2–4% and increases with maternal age, irrespective of any drug effect. Cohort studies indicate that this risk is increased to 4–12% in babies exposed to lithium, 11% in those exposed to valproate and 6% in those exposed to carbamazepine. Thus, the majority of women who conceive while taking these agents will deliver a normal baby. Lamotrigine has a slightly lower risk than the other anticonvulsants, while the risks with antipsychotics and antidepressants appear to be lower again. Smaller risks are, however, more difficult to quantify meaningfully.

If it were without risks, withdrawal of medication would often appear an appealing course of action. Unfortunately, pregnancy is not, as sometimes believed, a privileged period of low risk for mood disorder. Relapse may follow discontinuation of long-term treatment and can harm the mother–child relationship directly or via comorbid alcohol, drug or nicotine consumption. In addition, treating an acutely manic or depressed state in pregnancy may require a combination of medicines in higher doses than would be usual for maintenance.

Compromise treatment options include switching to alternatives associated with lower fetal risk prior to conception, or withdrawing some or all medication prior to conception and reintroducing it after the first trimester or immediately after birth or cessation of breastfeeding. Use of slow-release formulations twice or more times daily can minimize peak levels.

Women prescribed lithium, valproate, carbamazepine or lamotrigine during the first trimester should be told about prenatal diagnosis and offered maternal α-fetoprotein screening and a high-resolution ultrasound scan at 16–18 weeks' gestation. Folate supplementation is advised for all pregnant women and may reduce the increased risk of neural tube deficits associated particularly with carbamazepine and valproate.

Childbirth increases the risk of subsequent early manic and depressive relapse and must be a time for increased clinical vigilance on the part of patients, carers and clinicians.

## Neurotoxicity of maternal psychotropic medication after birth

Postnatal care. If women are taking medicines up to childbirth, vigilance in postnatal care is essential. Reports tend to be anecdotal but the mechanisms are potentially attributable to toxicity, withdrawal or a combination of factors. Benzodiazepines may depress neonatal respiration or cause drowsiness, hypotonia or withdrawal symptoms. Antipsychotics have been reported to cause EPS. Tricyclics have been reported to cause urinary retention and functional bowel obstruction. Lithium has been associated with thyroid goiter, hypotonia and cyanosis. Carbamazepine has caused neonatal bleeding. Antidepressants are associated with increased reports of jitteriness, poor feeding, crying and seizures.

Breastfeeding requires an understanding by mothers of the potential risks of toxicity to the neonate and the ongoing need for vigilance in their care. All drugs enter breast milk but the ratio between infant and maternal plasma levels varies greatly and the frequency of adverse effects is uncertain. It depends upon sporadic reports of, for example, toxicity due to lithium, hepatic dysfunction due to carbamazepine and thrombocytopenia or anemia attributed to valproate. In general, the risks to the infant are the same as those for any patient exposed to the medicine. Such risks must be balanced against the benefits of breastfeeding. Given its narrow therapeutic index, lithium is generally regarded as being a relative contraindication to breastfeeding because it is present in breast milk at 40% of the maternal serum concentration.

**Key points – long-term treatments**

- Long-term treatment with appropriate drugs is advocated from as early in the illness as is acceptable to the patient and family.
- In bipolar I disorder, lithium prevents relapse of mania. It is relatively less effective against depression but may reduce the risk of suicide.
- Quetiapine reduces the risk of relapse to mania and depression, as monotherapy or in combination with lithium or valproate.
- Olanzapine, aripiprazole and valproate may be as effective as lithium in the prevention of relapse to mania.
- Lamotrigine is more effective against depression than mania in long-term treatment.
- Carbamazepine is less effective than lithium.
- When the risk of a severe depressive relapse is high, antidepressants to which patients have shown an acute treatment response may, if appropriate, be continued long term, in combination with a drug showing long-term antimanic efficacy.
- Discontinuation of long-term treatment is not indicated when there is good clinical control of the illness.
- Successful long-term management often appears to require combination treatment. At present, there is little to guide practice, other than safety concerns and pragmatic outcomes in individual cases.
- The physical health of bipolar patients may be compromised by the choice of long-term medication; monitoring for cardiovascular risk factors must become a new focus, particularly in groups with high rates of obesity.
- Routine monitoring for metabolic risks and other toxicity is recommended for patients receiving long-term treatment.
- There is no simple rule to determine whether treatment should be stopped during pregnancy: a clinical judgment is required, weighing the risks and benefits with the patient's preferences and past history.

## Key references

Altshuler L, Kiriakos L, Calcagno J et al. The impact of antidepressant discontinuation versus antidepressant continuation on 1-year risk for relapse of bipolar depression: a retrospective chart review. *J Clin Psychiatry* 2001;62:612–16.

Austin MP, Mitchell PB. Use of psychotropic medications in breast-feeding women: acute and prophylactic treatment. *Aust N Z J Psychiatry* 1998;32:778–84.

Buse JB. Metabolic side effects of antipsychotics: focus on hyperglycemia and diabetes. *J Clin Psychiatry* 2002;63(suppl 4):37–41.

Cohen LS, Friedman JM, Jefferson JW et al. A re-evaluation of risk of in utero exposure to lithium. *JAMA* 1994;271:146–50.

Geddes JR, Carney SM, Davies C et al. Relapse prevention with antidepressant drug treatment in depressive disorders: a systematic review. *Lancet* 2003;361:653–61.

Goodwin FK, Fireman B, Simon GE et al. Suicide risk in bipolar disorder during treatment with lithium and divalproex. *JAMA* 2003;290: 1467–73.

Goodwin GM. Recurrence of mania after lithium withdrawal. Implications for the use of lithium in the treatment of bipolar affective disorder. *Br J Psychiatry* 1994; 164:149–52.

Greil W, Ludwig-Mayerhofer W, Erazo N et al. Lithium versus carbamazepine in the maintenance treatment of bipolar disorders – a randomised study. *J Affect Disord* 1997;43:151–61.

Marangell LB, Dennehy EB, Wisniewski SR et al. Case-control analyses of the impact of pharmacotherapy on prospectively observed suicide attempts and completed suicides in bipolar disorder: findings from STEP-BD. *J Clin Psychiatry* 2008;69:916–22.

Okuma T, Kishimoto A. A history of investigation on the mood stabilizing effect of carbamazepine in Japan. *Psychiatry Clin Neurosci* 1998; 52:3–12.

Prien RF, Kupfer DJ, Mansky PA et al. Drug therapy in the prevention of recurrences in unipolar and bipolar affective disorders. Report of the NIMH Collaborative Study Group comparing lithium carbonate, imipramine, and a lithium carbonate-imipramine combination. *Arch Gen Psychiatry* 1984;41:1096–104.

Smith S. Effects of antipsychotics on sexual and endocrine function in women: implications for clinical practice. *J Clin Psychopharmacol* 2003;23(3 suppl 1):S27–32.

Viguera AC, Whitfield T, Baldessarini RJ et al. Risk of recurrence in women with bipolar disorder during pregnancy: prospective study of mood stabilizer discontinuation. *Am J Psychiatry* 2007;164:1817–24.

Yatham LN, Kennedy SH, O'Donovan C et al. Canadian Network for Mood and Anxiety Treatments (CANMAT) guidelines for the management of patients with bipolar disorder: update 2007. *Bipolar Disord* 2006;8:721–39.

TABLE 7.1

**Medicines used for long-term treatment**

Additional information about medicines
For newer agents (the atypical antipsychotics), clinicians should refer to the SPC and emerging evidence. Unexpected adverse effects in bipolar patients should be reported to the relevant licensing authority. There is much accumulated experience to guide the use of lithium, but it is potentially

| | Lithium | Valproate |
|---|---|---|
| Significant contra-indications | • Renal impairment<br>• Complicated fluid or salt balance<br>• Acute myocardial infarction<br>• Myasthenia gravis<br>• Pregnancy | • Impairment of liver function<br>• Blood dyscrasia |
| Drug interactions | • Diuretics<br>• NSAIDs<br>• Carbamazepine<br>• Calcium channel blockers<br>• ACE inhibitors<br>• Metronidazole<br>• Neuroleptics | • Inhibits hepatic metabolism<br>• Increases levels of<br>  – Aspirin<br>  – Anticoagulants<br>  – Fatty acids<br>  – Lamotrogine<br>  – Ammonia |

toxic and litigation is possible if accepted procedures are not followed. Experience with anticonvulsants in bipolar patients is growing, but is already extensive in patients with epilepsy. If in doubt, consult the SPC or individual manufacturers for latest safety information.

| Carbamazepine | Lamotrigine |
|---|---|
| • Impairment of cardiac, renal or liver function<br>• Prior hematologic dyscrasia | • Impairment of liver function<br>• Renal impairment |
| • Induces CYP<br>• Reduces levels of<br>  – Antipsychotics<br>  – Lamotrigine<br>  – Oral contraceptives<br>  – Many others<br>• Level of carbamazepine may be increased when CYP blocked by:<br>  – Fluoxetine<br>  – Valproate<br>  – Histamine $H_2$ blockers<br>  – Erythromycin<br>  – Isoniazid<br>  – Propoxiphene<br>  – Calcium channel  blockers<br>• Carbamazepine + lithium may result in a rash | • Valproate reduces metabolism, so halve dose of lamotrigine<br><br>• Caution when using with carbamazepine<br>  – double doses may be required but side effects may be increased |

CONTINUED

TABLE 7.1 (CONTINUED)

| | Lithium | Valproate |
|---|---|---|
| Most common adverse effects | • Gastrointestinal irritation<br>• Sedation<br>• Tremor<br>• Other important effects:<br>– Weight gain<br>– Edema<br>– Acne<br>– Psoriasis<br>– Polyuria<br>– Polydipsia | • Tremor<br>• Dizziness<br>• Sedation<br>• Nausea/vomiting<br>• Gastrointestinal pain<br>• Headache<br>• Elevated LFTs |
| Most worrisome adverse effects | • Acute intoxication:<br>– Seizure<br>– Coma<br>– Death<br>• Intoxication sequelae:<br>– Renal<br>– Cardiac<br>– Central nervous system<br>• At therapeutic levels:<br>– Thyroid inhibition<br>– Renal dysfunction<br>– Arrhythmias<br>– Teratogenicity | • Marrow suppression<br>• Thrombocytopenia<br>• Prolongation of coagulation time<br>• Pancreatitis<br>• Hair loss<br>• Weight gain<br>• Teratogenicity |

| Carbamazepine | Lamotrigine |
| --- | --- |

- Dizziness
- Sedation
- Unsteady gait
- Incoordination
- Cognitive impairment
- Blurred vision/diplopia
- Elevated LFTs
- Gastrointestinal
  - Nausea
  - Anorexia
  - Pain

- Dizziness
- Ataxia
- Sedation
- Insomnia
- Nausea/vomiting

---

- Aplastic anemia
- Agranulocytosis
- Thrombocytopenia
- Hepatitis
- Skin adverse effects:
  - Rash (pruritic, erythematous)
  - Erythema multiforme or nodosum
  - Toxic epidermal necrolysis
  - Stevens–Johnson syndrome
- Hyponatremia
- Altered thyroid function
- Edema
- Arrhythmia, AV block
- Alopecia
- SLE
- Potential teratogen

- Stevens–Johnson syndrome
- Other important effects:
  - Rash
  - Blurred vision/diplopia
  - Esophagitis

CONTINUED

TABLE 7.1 (CONTINUED)

| | Lithium | Valproate |
|---|---|---|
| Initiating long-term treatment | *Pretreatment assessments*<br>• CBC<br>• Electrolytes<br>• Thyroid function tests<br>• Creatinine<br>• Urinalysis<br>• ECG if clinically indicated<br>*Initial dose regimen*<br>400 mg at night then titrate to the highest well-tolerated dose<br>*Usual maintenance dose*<br>800–1200 mg, but lower in the elderly | *Pretreatment assessments*<br>• CBC<br>• Platelets<br>• LFTs<br>*Initial dose regimen*<br>250–500 mg twice daily<br>Consider single dose at night<br>*Alternative rapid titration*<br>Day 1: single dose 20 mg/kg; day 2–4: continue split twice daily<br>Target level > 80 µg/mL<br>*During titration* consider serum valproate levels<br>Usual maintenance dose 1250 mg/day or more |
| Follow-up laboratory tests | • Serum lithium 3-monthly and every 12 months or when clinically indicated:<br>• Thyroid function tests<br>• Creatinine<br>• Urinalysis<br>• CBC (expect neutrophilia) | • CBC and LFTs every 6–12 months or if clinically indicated |

| Carbamazepine | Lamotrigine |
|---|---|
| *Pretreatment assessments* | *Pretreatment assessments* |
| • CBC | • No laboratory tests required |
| • Platelets | *Initial dose regimen* |
| • LFTs | 25 mg/day for 2 weeks, then |
| • Urinalysis | 50 mg/day for 2 weeks, then |
| *Initial dose regimen* | increase each week by |
| 400 mg at night | 100 mg to usual maintenance |
| Titrate to clinical response | dose |
| (not to specific serum level) | *During titration:* no laboratory |
| over 7–14 days | tests required |
| *Usual maintenance dose* | *Usual maintenance dose* |
| 800 mg or more | 200–400 mg/day |
| | If added to valproate, halve |
| | dose |
| | If added to carbamazepine, |
| | double dose (note that side |
| | effects may increase) |
| | |
| • Consider regular CBC and LFTs | Potentially useful (especially |
| | if lamotrigine is given |
| | concurrently with drug |
| | that alters metabolism) |
| | • Serum levels |
| | • LFTs |

CONTINUED

TABLE 7.1 (CONTINUED)

| | Lithium | Valproate |
|---|---|---|
| Points to cover in patient education | *Expect (one or more)* <br> • Mild tremor <br> • Thirst <br> • Gastrointestinal irritation <br> • Sedation <br> *Report to doctor* <br> • Moderate tremor <br> • Slurred speech <br> • Muscle twitching <br> • Change in fluid balance <br> • Memory impairment <br> • Rash <br> • Edema <br> *Discuss* <br> • Laboratory rationale <br> • Weight control <br> • Importance of sodium <br> • Potential teratogenicity | *Expect* <br> • Sedation <br> • Tremor <br> • Gastrointestinal symptoms <br> *Report to doctor* <br> • Easy bruising <br> • Abdominal swelling <br> • Rash <br> • Jaundice <br> • Edema (facial) <br> *Discuss* <br> • Weight control program <br> • Common drug interactions <br> • Potential teratogenicity <br> • Use of vitamins/minerals (folate, selenium, zinc) |

ACE, angiotensin-converting enzyme; AV, atrioventricular; CBC, complete blood count; CNS, central nervous system; CYP, cytochrome P450; ECG, electrocardiogram; GI, gastrointestinal; $H_2$, histamine $H_2$; LFTs, liver function tests; MI, myocardial infarction; NSAID, non-steroidal anti-inflammatory drug; SLE, systemic lupus erythematosus; SPC, summary of product characteristics.

| Carbamazepine | Lamotrigine |
|---|---|
| *Expect* | *Expect (transiently)* |
| • Sedation | • Insomnia/sedation |
| • Gastrointestinal symptoms | • Nausea |
| • Lightheadedness | • Dizziness |
| *Report to doctor* | *Report to doctor* |
| • Rash | • Rash |
| • Jaundice | • Easy bruising |
| • Incoordination | • Abdominal swelling |
| • Irregular heartbeat | • Jaundice |
| • Facial edema | • Edema (facial) |
| *Discuss* | *Discuss* |
| • Importance of weight control program | • Common drug interactions |
| • Common drug interactions | • Use of vitamins/minerals (folate, selenium, zinc) |
| • Potential teratogenicity | |
| • Use of vitamins/minerals (folate, selenium, zinc) | |

The foregoing chapters have painted a broad overview of bipolar disorder: its nature as a clinical problem, our attempts to classify it and understand the causes, and, most importantly, how we think it is best treated. We hope we have made the case for a scientific approach to psychiatry based on what has worked for other medical problems such as diabetes and heart disease. We believe that this approach is starting to work for bipolar disorder too.

The discoveries that we expect to make a major difference in the coming years fall under three headings: genetics, neuroscience and treatment trials. We think they may change practice for the better, and so we hope patients and clinicians will support efforts to get the clinical work done. Making a case for progress may seem superfluous, but overzealous ethical rule-making on the one hand, and an anti-science populism on the other, threaten research in all the areas that we believe will be most important for bipolar disorder, particularly in Europe.

## Genetics

Psychiatric geneticists have, perhaps for too long, promised much and delivered little. The Human Genome Project, and the advances in technology that it has stimulated, mean that we now stand on the threshold of understanding the molecular genetic associations of bipolar disorder. These associations are likely to inform our understanding of the etiology at every possible level. At its simplest, this could transform diagnosis because we will quickly see how far our phenotypic subtypes are reflected in genetic variation. It will also provide an array of treatment targets with as yet unknown connections to the phenomenology of bipolar disorders. Perhaps it will reveal important secrets about brain development and function.

Genetic variation may also operate to modify environmental effects and treatment. Thus, pharmacogenetics may come to dominate how we choose between different pharmacological and non-pharmacological treatments, because some genotypes may favor a particular response to treatment more than others. We expect that the heterogeneity of response, which we can now simply witness, will be illuminated by genotyping. It will therefore inform how we select the most effective management plan for individual patients. The major threat to this kind of development is already clear: the numbers of genes involved are very large and individual genetic effects very small. The challenge is to translate the small certainties of the current genetic projects into better measures of function.

## Neuroscience

Neuroscience offers an integrated and essentially singular view of how the brain works, although it draws on the expertise of traditionally separate disciplines. Advances in cognitive psychology, psychopharmacology, brain imaging and cell biology are highly likely to change our understanding of what underlies mood and emotion in health. This improved understanding of brain/mind function will inevitably break down the current conceptual barriers to understanding psychiatric disease. It is particularly important that we identify the functional pathology of bipolar disorder, as this is likely to transform how we define outcomes in treatment studies and our understanding of how treatments work. Current strategies emphasize the treatment and prevention of syndromal relapse. Disabling aspects of long-term outcome, such as chronic depressive symptoms or enduring neurocognitive impairment, may become important therapeutic targets in the future.

## Improvements in treatment

Finally, we wish to see improvements in treatment. We have emphasized how care can be enhanced by commonsense, structured psychological interventions and we expect to see further modest, but important, progress in this direction. However, bipolar disorder is a strongly biologically determined disease and we hope to see more effective use of drugs in the coming years. This may come from the neurobiology – from translation of basic findings to the clinic – and improved patient selection. There is currently an important gap between clinical trials showing average benefits in unselected populations of bipolar I and II patients and the individual patient we try to treat optimally in the clinic.

Individuals sometimes do much better than average on individual treatments or combinations of treatments; others do much worse. In neither case do we really know why, and yet that is the knowledge we would prize above all, and so would our patients.

In conclusion, we have written this book at a time when something approaching a consensus has emerged among clinicians treating bipolar disorder. The accumulation of new evidence – the fast facts provided here – has made this possible. Consensus implies agreeing on what we know and also, sometimes more interestingly, on what we need to know. As we hope to have made plain, there are no grounds for complacency, but the research agenda is an exciting one. Only a commitment to clinical research in psychiatry from funding agencies, health services, industry, clinicians and patients will deliver the knowledge we need for innovation and improvement.

**Key references**

Dawson GR, Goodwin GM. Experimental medicine in psychiatry. *J Psychopharmacol* 2005;19:565–6.

Flint J, Munafò MR. The endophenotype concept in psychiatric genetics. *Psychol Med* 2007;37:163–80.

Goodwin GM, Geddes JR. What is the heartland of psychiatry? *Br J Psychiatry* 2007; 191:189–91.

Insel TR, Charney DS. Research on major depression: strategies and priorities. *JAMA* 2003;289:3167–8.

Meyer-Lindenberg A, Weinberger DR. Intermediate phenotypes and genetic mechanisms of psychiatric disorders. *Nat Rev Neurosci* 2006;7:818–27.

Watson JD. Genes and politics. *J Mol Med* 1997;75:624–36.

# Useful resources

## UK
### British Association for Psychopharmacology
36 Cambridge Place, Hills Road
Cambridge CB2 1NS
Tel: +44 (0)1223 321268
www.bap.org.uk

### Electronic Medicines Compendium
List of all licensed medications available in the UK
www.emc.medicines.org.uk

### MDF The BiPolar Organisation
Castle Works, 21 St George's Road
London SE1 6ES
Toll-free: 0808 802 1983
www.mdf.org.uk

### Mind
Leading mental health charity in England and Wales
15–19 Broadway
London E15 4BQ
Tel: +44 (0)20 8519 2122
Mind*info*Line: 0845 766 0163
info@mind.org.uk
www.mind.org.uk

### Netdoctor
Information and news on depression, discussion forums and chatrooms, support services and an 'ask the expert' service
www.netdoctor.co.uk/depression

### NHS Evidence – mental health
A specialist library at the Health Information Resources website
www.library.nhs.uk

### PsychNet-UK
Mental health and psychology directory
Toll-free: 0845 122 8622
www.psychnet-uk.com

## USA
### American Psychiatric Association
1000 Wilson Boulevard, Suite 1825
Arlington, VA 22209-3901
Tel: +1 703 907 7300
apa@psych.org
www.psych.org

### American Psychological Association
750 First Street NE
Washington, DC 20002-4242
Toll-free: 1 800 374 2721
Tel: +1 202 336 5500
www.apa.org

## Depression and Bipolar Support Alliance
US patient organization with many useful links
730 N. Franklin Street, Suite 501
Chicago, IL 60654-7225
Toll-free: 1 800 826 3632
www.dbsalliance.org

## Massachusetts General Hospital Bipolar Clinic & Research Program
Information on research and treatment, including the STEP-BD program (www.stepbd.org), and many useful links
50 Staniford St, Suite 580
Boston, MA 02114
Tel: +1 617 726 5855
www.manicdepressive.org

## Medscape
A large US database linked to other useful medical databases
www.medscape.com/psychiatry

## National Alliance on Mental Illness
3803 N. Fairfax Dr., Ste. 100
Arlington, VA 22203
Helpline: 1 800 950 6264
Tel: +1 703 524 7600
www.nami.org

## International
### Balance NZ
New Zealand bipolar and depression network
www.balance.org.nz

### Beyond Blue
Australian national depression initiative
www.beyondblue.org.au

### Bipolar Significant Others
Information and support for friends and family of adults with bipolar disorder
www.bpso.org

### Child and Adolescent Bipolar Foundation
Information and support for families raising children with, or at risk of, bipolar disorder
www.bpkids.org

### Pendulum
An online support group for individuals with bipolar disorder
www.pendulum.org

### Society for Manic Depression
Comprehensive resource directory on depression
www.societymd.org

# Disclosures

The authors are conscious of current controversies about conflict of interest in scientific and especially medical writing. We regard ourselves as holding independent opinions and we have expressed them as honestly as we can in this book. However, like most, if not all, responsible adults in professional positions, we have potential conflicts of interest. By conflicts of interest we mean relationships, allegiances or hostilities to particular groups, organizations or interests, which could excessively influence our judgments or actions. The issue is obviously most sensitive when such interests are private and/or may result in personal gain. We have identified a hierarchy of such possible interests in declaring ours.

### Guy Goodwin
- I own shares in P1vital, a company with interests in the area of psychopharmacology.
- I have acted within the last year as a paid consultant to AstraZeneca, Bristol-Myers Squibb, Lundbeck, Roche, Servier and Wyeth. I have also advised GlaxoSmithKline, Janssen and Lilly in the past.
- I have acted as an expert witness for Pfizer and Lilly.
- I hold or have held agreements with Sanofi to supply Depakote for an independent clinical trial and with Servier to conduct experimental medicine research.
- I have accepted many paid speaking engagements in industry-supported symposia.
- I have occasionally accepted travel or hospitality unrelated to a speaking engagement from a pharmaceutical company.
- My primary employment is with Oxford University and the National Health Service in England.

### Gary Sachs
- My family has a substantial ownership interest in Concordant Raters Systems, LLC. I hold patent on systems tools invented for training

and monitoring raters in the using of rating scales in clinical research studies.

- Neither I nor my family has any other patents or inventions nor own any company with interests in the area of psychopharmacology.
- I have never accepted a personal retainer from any company with an interest in psychopharmacology.
- I have acted within the past year as a paid advisory board member or consultant to Abbott Laboratories, AstraZeneca, Bristol-Myers Squibb, Forest Laboratories, GlaxoSmithKline, Janssen, Lilly, Pfizer, Repligen, Sanofi Aventis, Sepracor, Takeda and Wyeth. In the past, I have also advised Elan, Memory Pharmaceuticals and Solvay.
- I currently conduct research studies funded by the National Institute of Mental Health and Repligen.
-  I am a member of the speakers' bureau or have given lectures or symposia sponsored by Abbott, AstraZeneca, Bristol-Myers Squibb, GlaxoSmithKline, Janssen, Lilly, Memory Pharmaceutical, Pfizer, Sanofi-Aventis and Wyeth.
- My primary employment is with Massachusetts General Hospital and Harvard University in the USA.

# Appendix: Generic and brand names of drugs

| Generic names | US brand names | UK brand names |
|---|---|---|
| **Drugs used in the treatment of patients with bipolar disorder** | | |
| Aripiprazole | Abilify | Abilify |
| Asenapine | Saphris | Not yet available |
| Bupropion | Wellbutrin Zyban | Zyban |
| Carbamazepine | Atretol Carbatrol Epitol Tegretol Equetro | Teril Retard Tegretol |
| Chlorpromazine | Thorazine | Largactil |
| Citalopram | Celexa | Cipramil |
| Clonazepam | Klonopin | Rivotril |
| Clozapine | Clozaril | Clozaril |
| Escitalopram | Lexapro | Cipralex |
| Fluoxetine | Prozac | Prozac |
| Fluvoxamine | Luvox | Faverin |
| Gabapentin | Neurontil | Neurontin |
| Haloperidol | Haldol | Dozic Haldol Serenace |
| Lamotrigine | Lamictal | Lamictal |
| Lithium (carbonate/citrate) | Eskalith Eskalith CR Lithobid | Camcolit Li-liquid Liskonum Priadel |
| Lorazepam | Ativan | Ativan |
| Moclobemide | – | Manerix |
| Olanzapine | Zyprexa | Zyprexa |

CONTINUED

| Generic names | US brand names | UK brand names |
| --- | --- | --- |
| Oxcarbazepine | Trileptal | Trileptal |
| Paliperidone | Invega | Invega |
| Paroxetine | Paxil | Seroxat |
| Phenelzine | Nardil | Nardil |
| Quetiapine | Seroquel | Seroquel |
| Risperidone | Risperdal | Risperdal |
| Sertraline | Zoloft | Lustral |
| Trancylpromine | Parnate | Parnate |
| Valproate | Depakene Depakote | Depakote |
| Ziprasidone | Geodon | Not available in UK |

**Other drugs referred to in the text**

| | | |
| --- | --- | --- |
| Amphetamine | Adderal Dexedrine Focalin | Dexedrine |
| Levodopa | Atamet Sinemet | Madopar Sinemet |
| Topiramate | Topamax | Topamax |

# Index

113

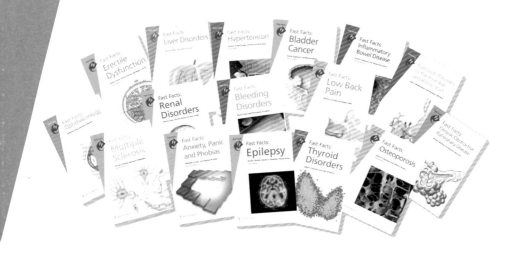